Any angel has t[o]

To live twice

THE ART OF KILLING

MARILYN MONROE

MURDER VERSION 1-2-3

Third serial book

Dr. Marilyn Monroe

A Honorary. Doctor degree

PhD & MBMD & D.A.M.

Dr. Marilyn. Norma Monroe. Is Marilyn Monroe at her present life. Bringing an assemblage of Memories and evidence around her past, present life and death, for the benefit of an opening of an investigation, around her murder case, occurred between the 4-5 of August 1962. Dr. Marilyn will celebrate her reborn in each 6 of May.

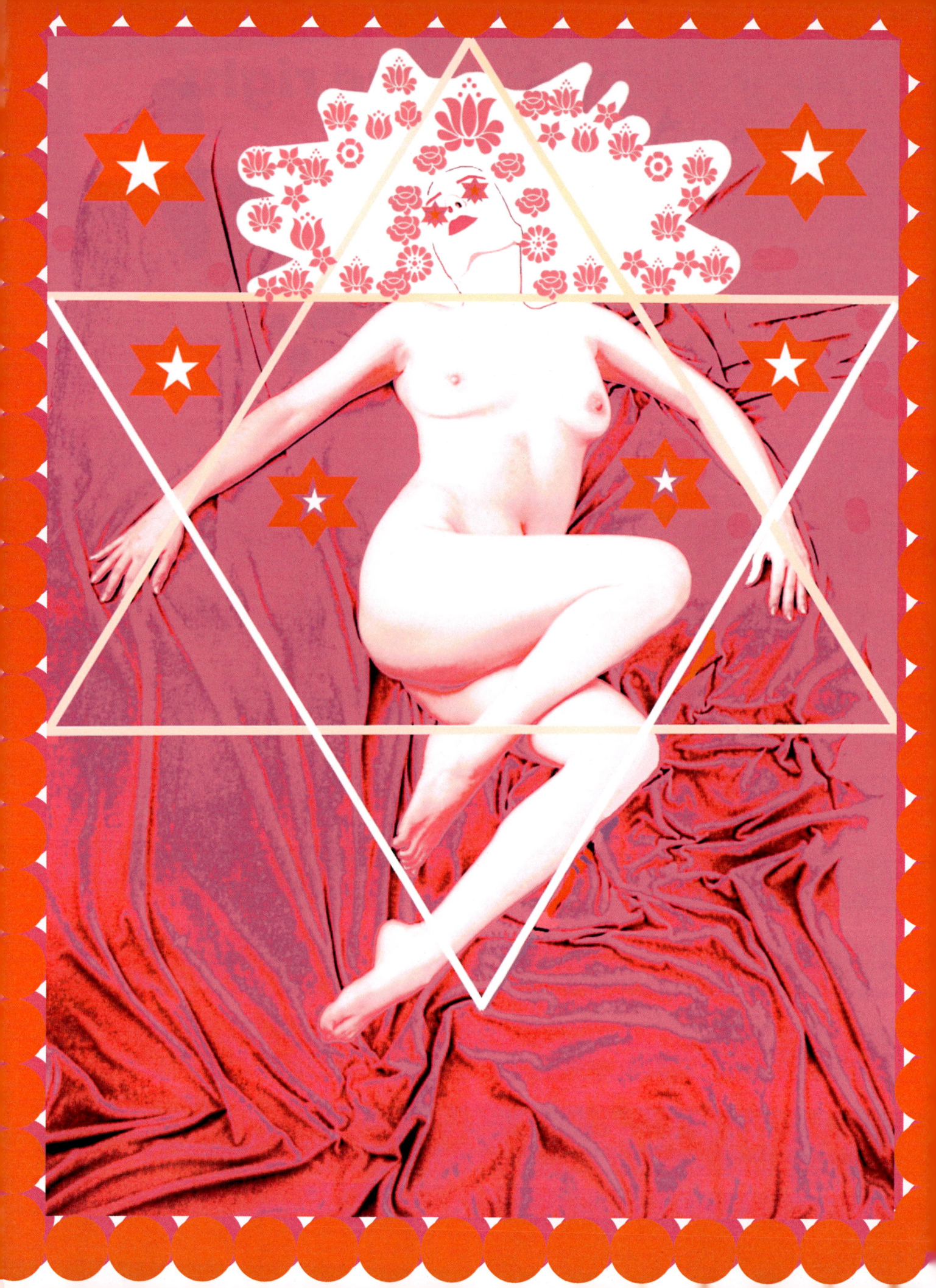

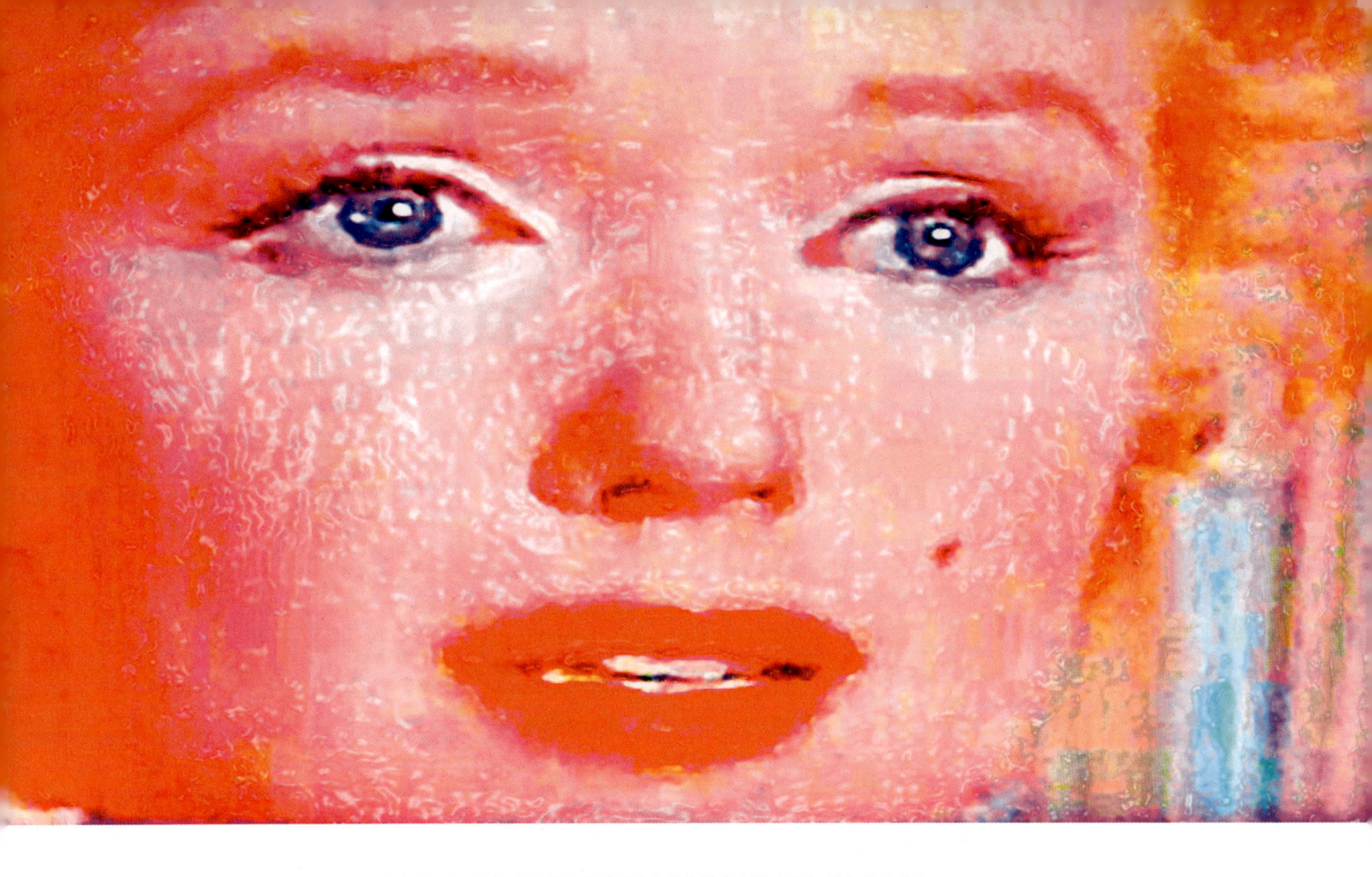

THIS BOOK, FIRST EDITION PUBLISHED IN 2016

The front and back cover: photography: Dr. Marilyn Monroe

Model Self-portrait. Painting: Dr. Marilyn Monroe

Produces. Grammatical edit. Graphics and layout book. Cover Design: Dr. Marilyn Monroe

The book includes: writing, poetry, paintings, modeling. Photography

All the photos and images are going toward a process by using Adobe Photoshop and or paint.net

Created by: Dr. Marilyn Norma Jean. Monroe. Copyright © 1976 - 2016 All rights reserved.

My legal advisor: Dr. Sarah Present. Adv. Debbi Aharonov. Literary advisor: Amira Morag. Photographs: Ofer Frohlich. Moti Dahan. Yoval Devir. Nir Mobdaly

Uzi Amir. Uri Akerman. Rafael Nagary. Oren Lavie. Carmit Nahum.

The font made with the blessing. www.fontsquirrel.com

The editing made with the blessing help of www.gingersoftware.com

Printed by CreateSpace. www.CreateSpace.com/TITLEID. Amazon.com Company.

Image 1 page 1. Magen David shield. Model. Painter: Dr. Marilyn. Photograph: Ofer Frohlich

290

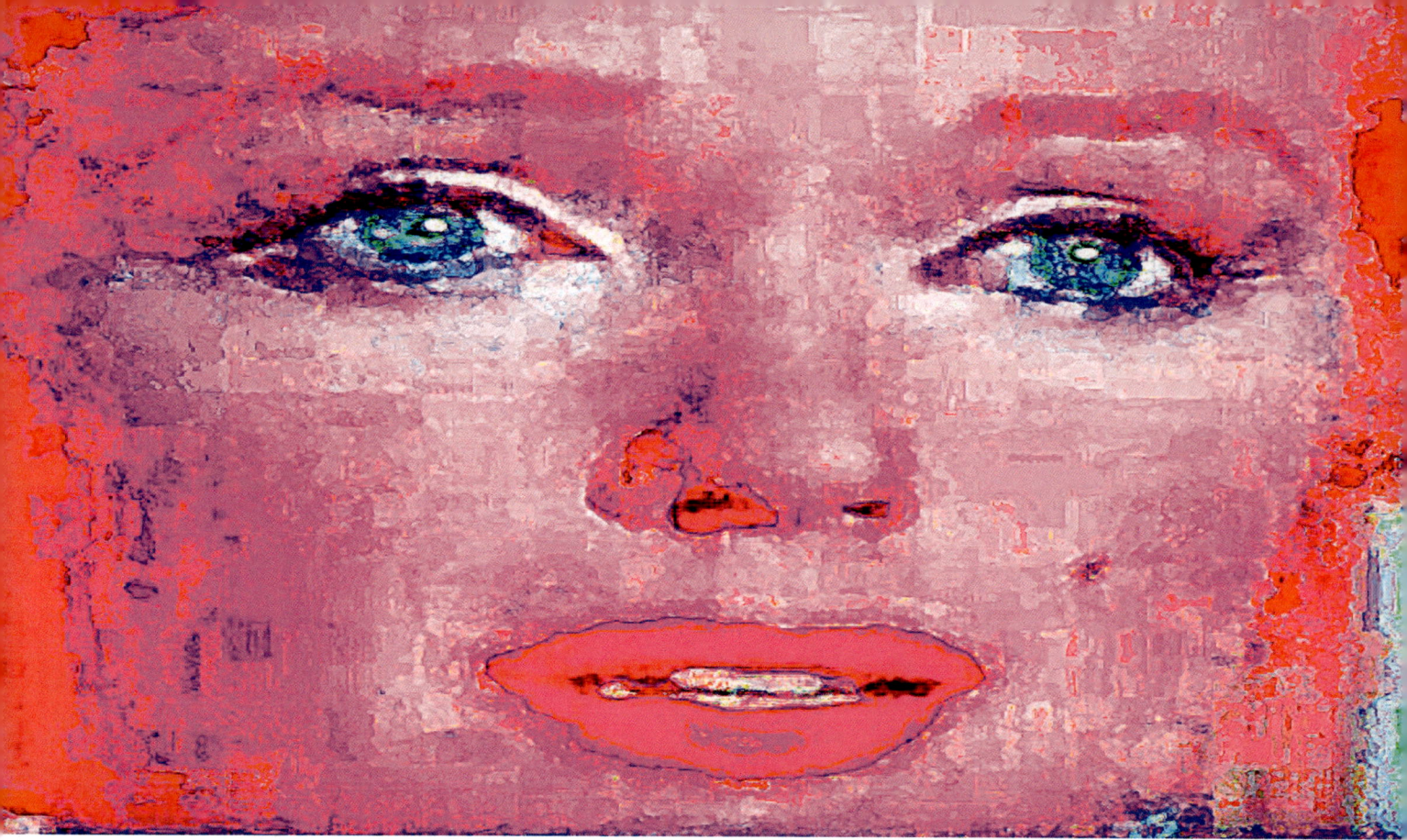

This comes back book process of conception based upon a deep life time investigation, I am doing around my case from the year 1976. In that year I had begun writing notes and especial diaries on the daily basis, since my past life time and my murder was running after me into the present. I used to see in my vision with my eyes open many scenes from my Marilyn Monroe life, all my comeback books are grounded in the materials I wrote inside of my diaries, Around the ages 10, at this present life, start to paint portray of a nude art as I did in my past. Some of the images inside of this book had started 40 years ago to build upwards. At the age 15 years old, I stood fully naked in front of a camera with no issue, since I used to do it in my past. This book is a summary of all the extremely arduous work I had performed along this last 51 years, around my comeback. I know some people will try to copy the info I exhibit in this book. Please take into consideration, you will have to stand in court and prove this info and ideas are yours, that my identity I was reborn with is yours. No one can be me but me.

**This book is deposited maintenance and protected
In a few copy right companies around the world
One of them is the USA Congress copyright company**

WARNING! COPYING PROHIBITION ENFORCED. WE WILL PROSECUTE ALL INTERNET THEFT OF OUR COPYRIGHTED MATERIAL. DO NOT COPY OUR TEXT OR IMAGES WITHOUT OUR PERMISSION. WE'RE CRACKING DOWN ON INTERNET PIRACY. IF YOU COPY OUR CONTENT. STEAL OUR CONTENT OR IMAGES, WE'LL STEAL YOUR HAPPINESS. NEVER RE-POST OUR MATERIAL ON YOUR WEBSITE OR BLOG. Dr. Marilyn. Norma Jean Monroe. Adit. Daniel. Is the sole and exclusive owner of this book and any of its content include written and images photos and painting. NO COPYING AND/OR DOWNLOADING AND/OR MAKING ANY COMMERCIAL AND/OR PERSONAL USE OF THIS BOOK OR ANY OF ITS CONTENTS FOR ANY PURPOSE WHATSOEVER, INCLUDING, BUT WITHOUT LIMITATION TO ANY REVERSE ENGINEERING, SPY SOFTWARE ETC. IS ALLOWED, This Book is for a personal private use only. No commercial use is allowed of any kind, of any part, idea, or info. Without the prior written approval of Dr. Adit Marilyn. Norma Jean Monroe.

**YOU AND ME
ARE THE ANGELS
THAT HAVE
THE RIGHT
TO LIVE
TWICE**

**Since the lord
Had created us
By his wisdom
With his
Unconditional

Love**

Image 2 page 5. Self-portrait. Model. Painter: Dr. Marilyn Monroe.

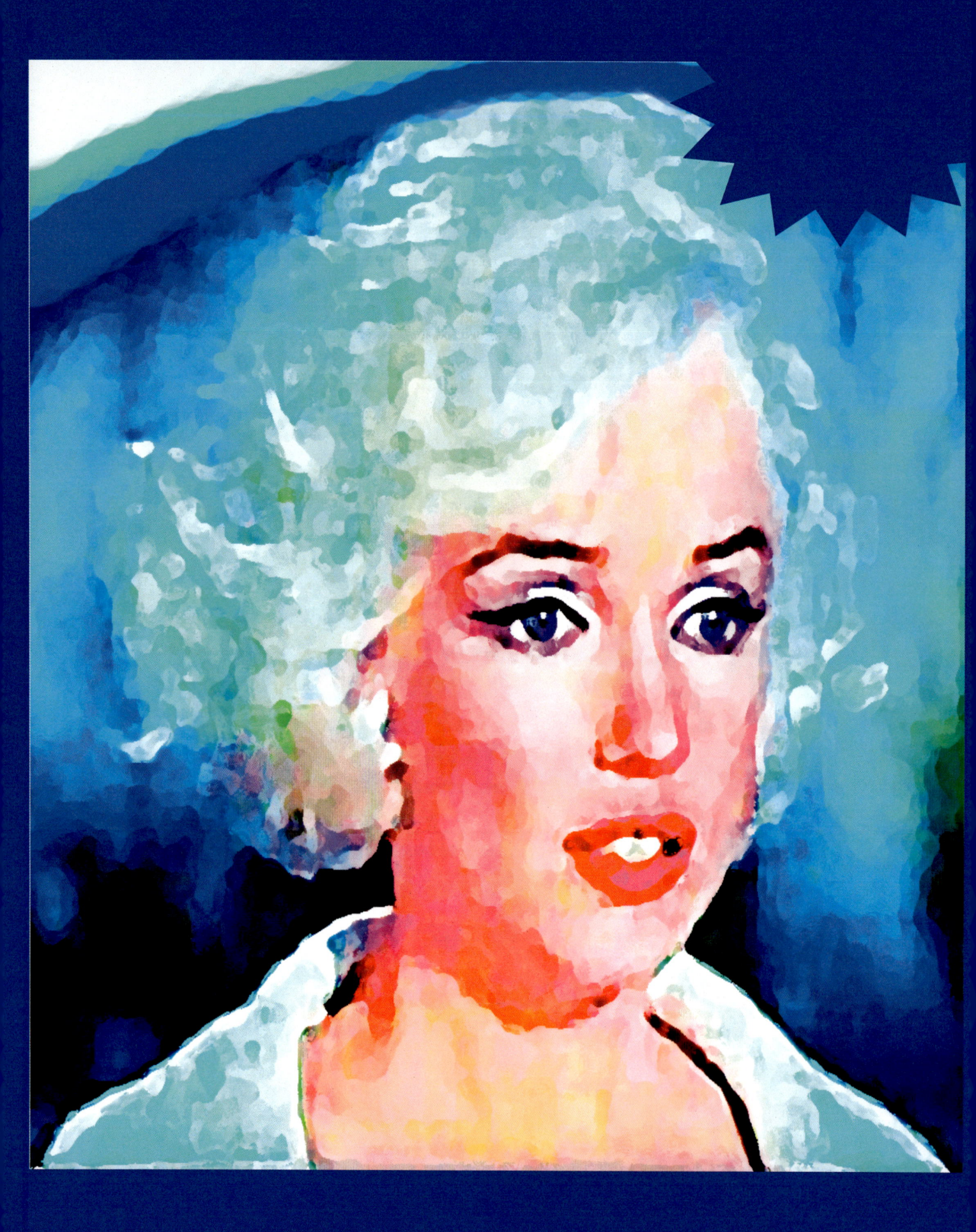

CONTENTS

CHAPTERS	PAGES
47. A SOUL REQUEST MR. LEONARDO DICAPRIO. MR. DONALD TRUMP. MRS YAEL. MRS. OPRAH WINFREY.	300
48. ONE. THE MAFIA BOYS	304
49. TWO. BABY GIRLS AND	308
50. THREE. JACKLIN WHERE ARE MY BABYS	312
51. FOUR. THE ART OF KILLING MARILYN VER 1	316
52. FIVE. MARILYN ORGANS	320
53. SIX. THE BEAUTY AND THE BEAST	324
54. SEVEN. MY SEX ORAL VIDEO	328
55. EIGHT. SEX WEAKEND WITH 100 MEN	332
56. NINE. THE HUNTED SOUL	338
57. TEN. LAST WEAKEND WITH MARILYN	342
58. ELEVEN. THE PRINCE AND MY HEAD STATU	348
59. TWELVE. DREAMS COME TURH. THE WISHFULL PRINCE	352
60. THIRTEEN. THE SHINING STAR INSIDE OF THE BLACK HOLE	356
61. FOURTEEN. MARILYN LAST SUPPER	362
62. FIFTEEN. ELECTRA COMPLEX AT THE RED FLAGS	370
63. SIXSTEEN. THE TEN COMMANDS	372
64. SEVENTEEN. JACKIE FANS – A SPELL MURDER VER 2	378

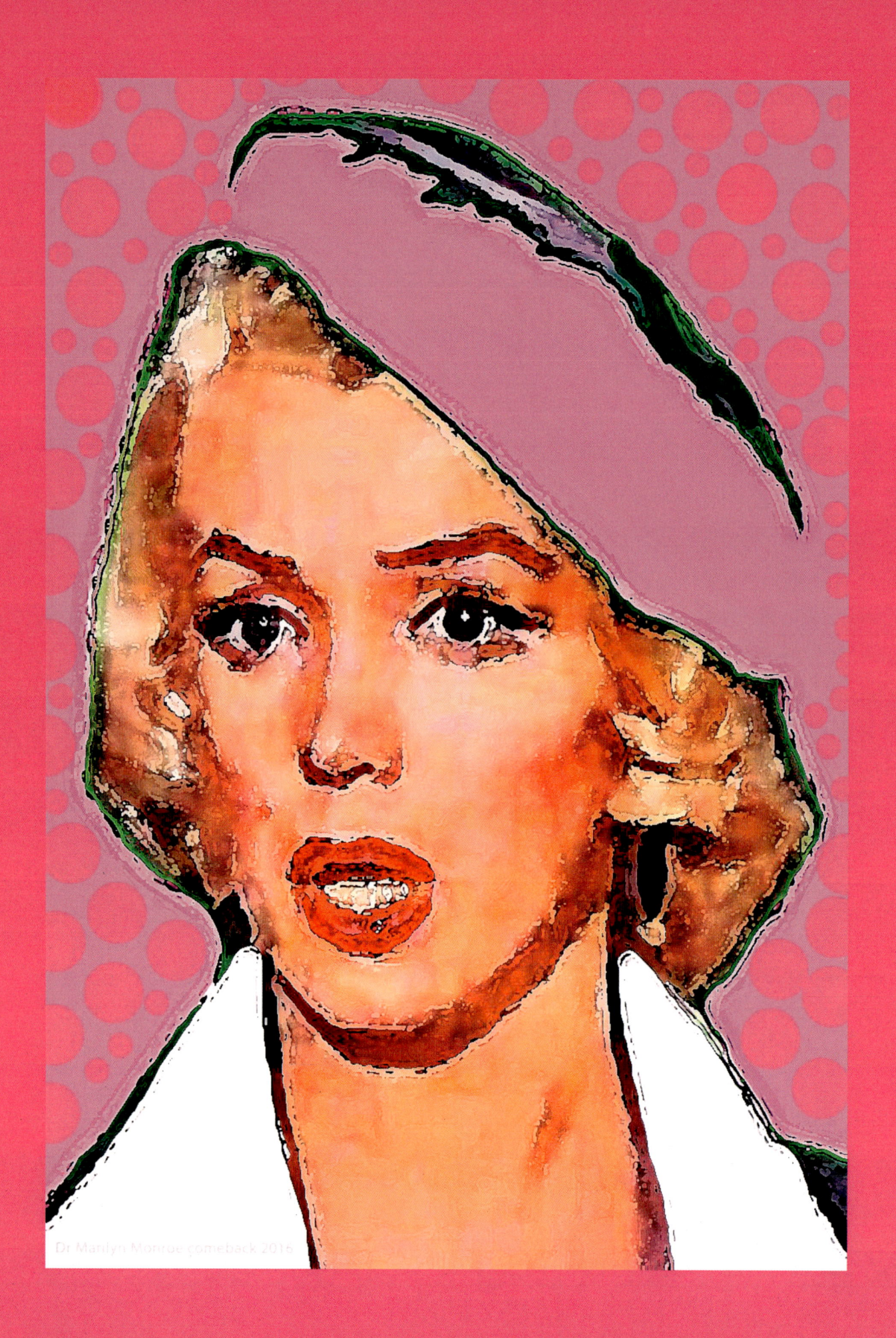

Dr Marilyn Monroe comeback 2016

WELCOM
TO THE COMEBACK
OF THE ONLY
MARILYN MONROE
INTO THE PRESENT

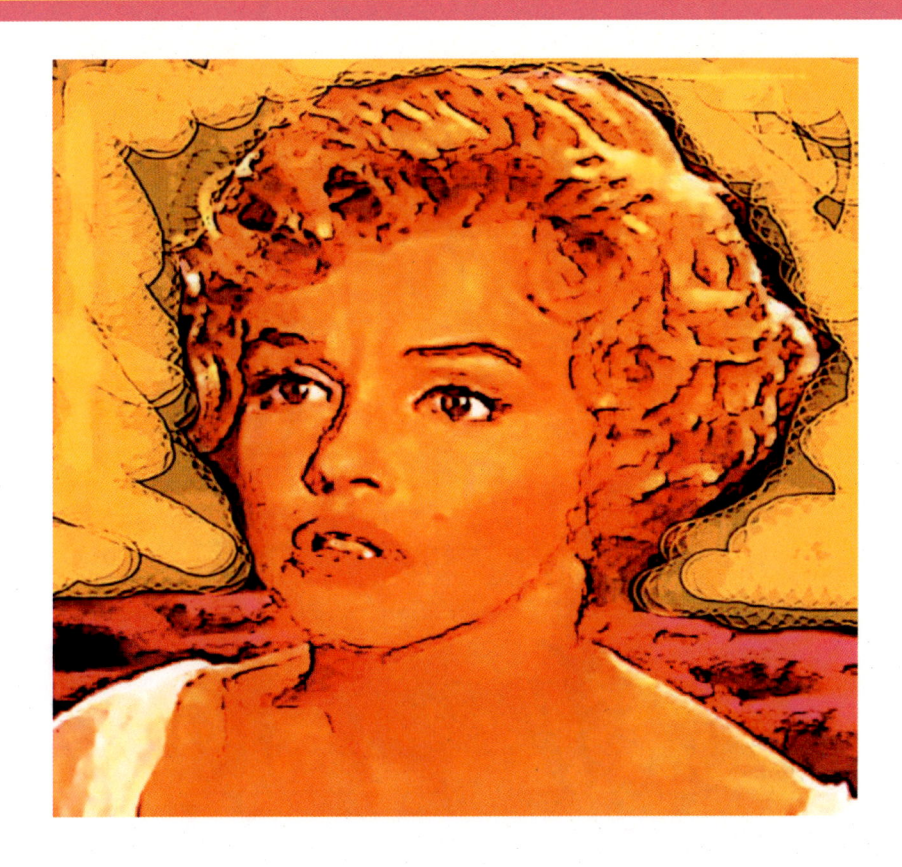

Image 6 page 15. David violin. Model. Painter: Dr. Marilyn Monroe. Photographer: Ofer Frohlich

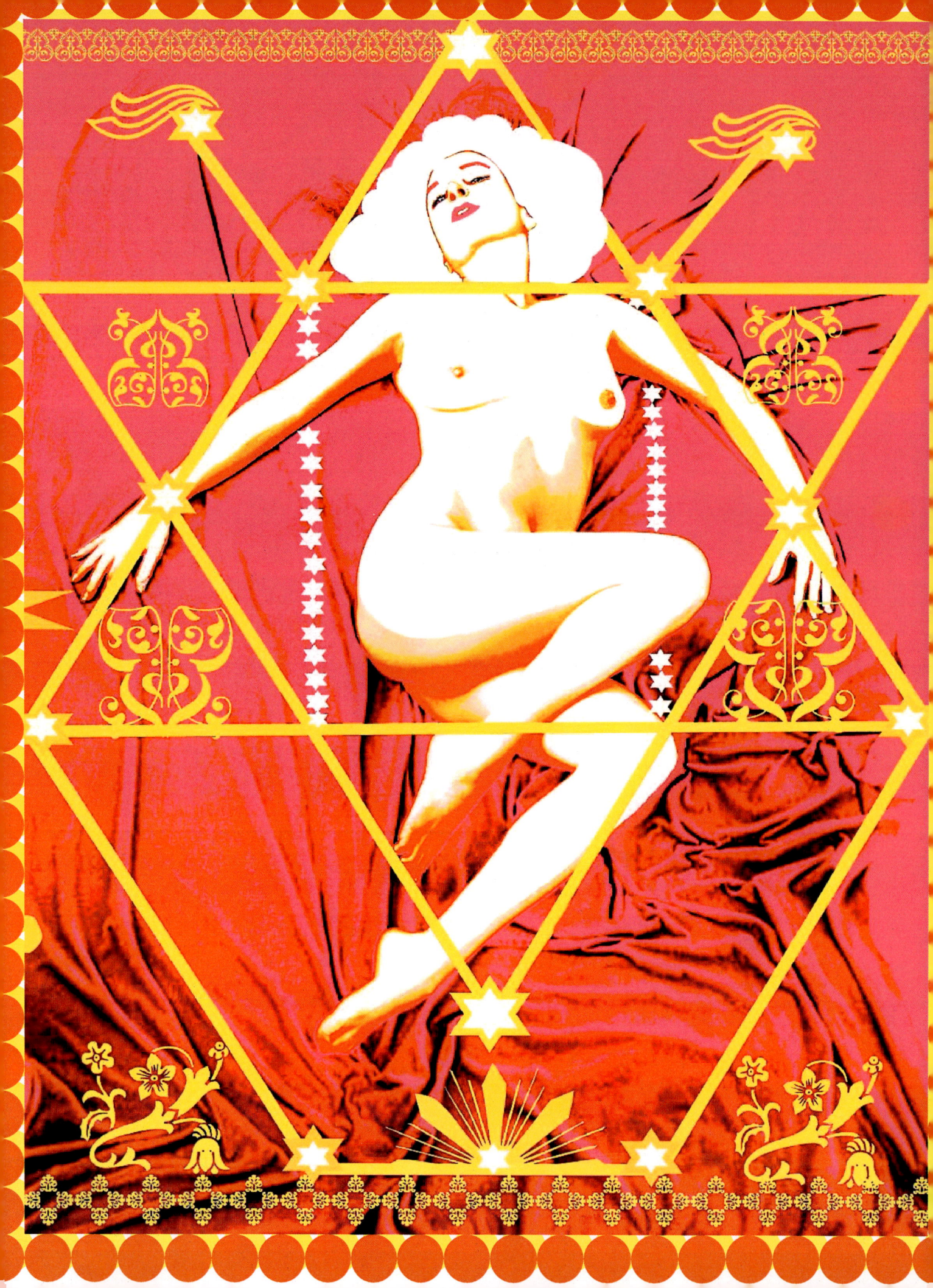

THE ITALIAN CHRISTIAN. JEWISH MAFIA COCKS

I HAD TO COME BACK

TO SHOW YOU THE WAY OUT

OF YOUR LIES

BELIVE IT OR NOT

YOUR COCKS DOESN'T COUNT

UNLESS IT'S COMES WITH

A WISE BRAIN. A BIG SOUL

AND A BIG WARM HEART

Image 129 page 277. Any angel had the right to live. Red. Model. Painter: Dr. Marilyn M. Photographer: Ofer Frohlich

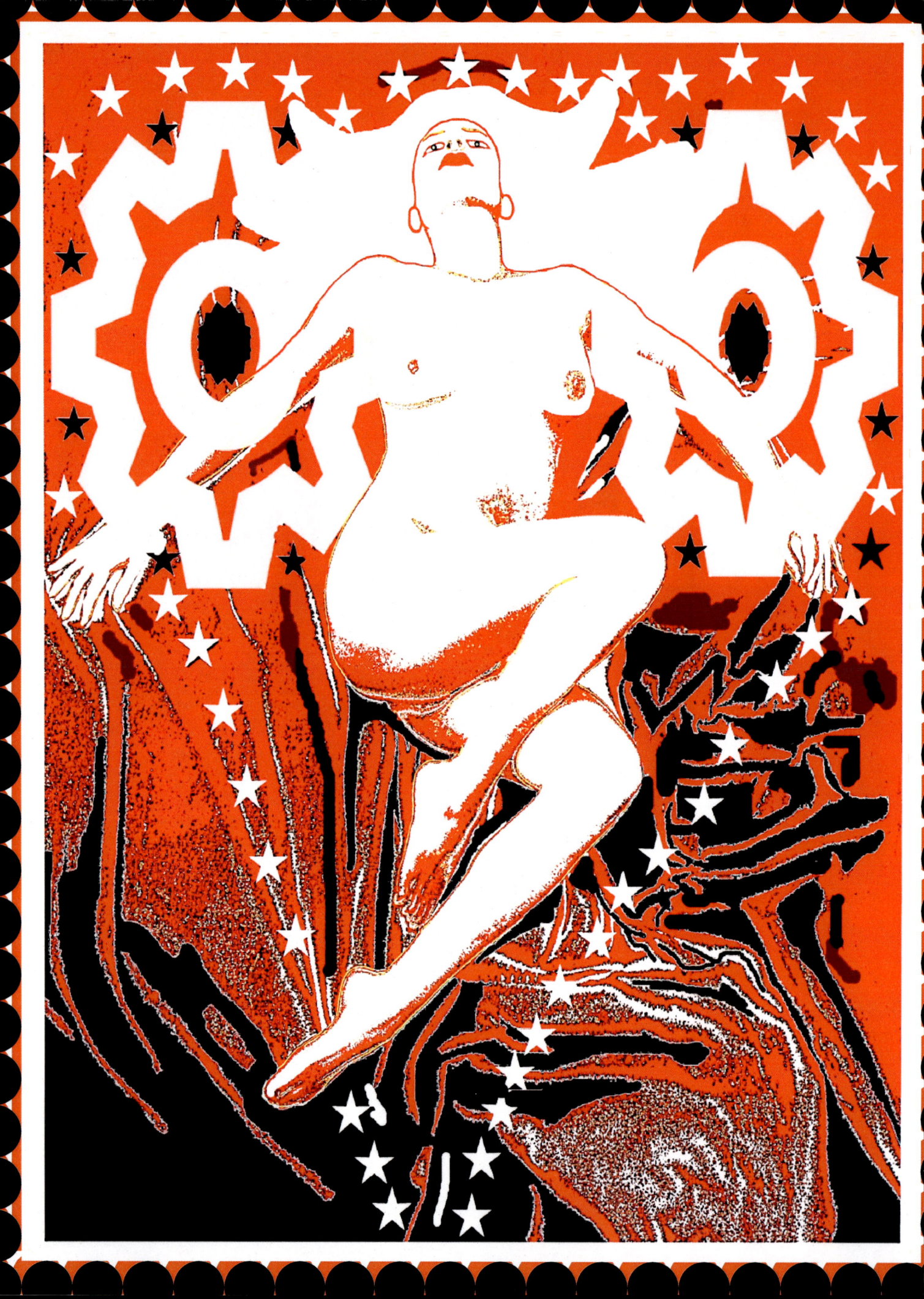

A soul request from Leonardo DiCaprio

Hello. Mr. Leonardo DiCaprio. A legendary actor. Your soul is from the line of Indigo diamond crystal souls. The fact you own a phenomenal talent, part of humanity can't cope with, which lead to the fact they couldn't give you the Oscar until today. This lack of ability to fully give a full credit for your phenomenal wisdom and diamond brain, is the same lack of ability I face until today, by the lack of ability, humanity got, which make them sees in me just a " a beautiful sex symbol". Side by side to it, they can't face the fact I used to own a phenomenal diamond brain. Most of humanity can't cope with the fact, my brain was in charge of my phenomenal Marilyn Monroe performance. One more characteristic you own, which shows you are an Indigo child, which is the fact, you know how to become as one person, with the characteristic you are playing in films, as well the fact, you care so much for mankind and the children living on this planet, by being influenced by the environment and climate change, these are the subjects indigo crystal children are taking care of the part you played as the boy suffering from a mental retardation in the film "What's Eating Gilbert, is very resemble to what I had to face with my mother Gladys and her mental health illness. The fact you are acting as the main role in the file "Titanic" is one more point which precedes me to think you will be able to understand things about my case others are blind to determine. I conceive I was before my late life as Marilyn Monroe, one of the victims with died on that ship. Since along all my childhood I used to dream about this drowning over and over once more, it was a regular horror dream which was waking me at nights. The fact you were playing in the "Titanic" a young artist a painter. The fact you are being called on the public figure of the famous legendary artist, Mr. Leonardo DA Vinci, which was the Indigo genius human of the ancient times. I trust you may be his reincarnation of his soul and your mother when she was seeing his paintings while being pregnant with you, I think her soul had felt it. Since you as DA Vinci both got the same ability to investigate deeper into the heart and essence behind things, bring the naked truth out, as I get along. This is the main reason why I, which was growing in this present life as an artist, my art today is grounded and being influenced from the age 10 when I start to go deeper into their plastic arts, until today on Leonardo DA Vinci arts. Therefore, I trust, you will be one of not many, who will possess the power, to recognize me, as the original Marilyn Monroe at my present life. I don't possess the same look I used to, but my soul, which is all I could take with me while living earth in 5 of August 1962 after being murder is here. I am about to ask from you two soul request: to help take care for my artistic legacy I own today, part of being exhibited along this book. if I will die ahead of my time again, since I live in Tel - Aviv, in Israel, my life is under a constant everyday risk and a terror danger. I can never be sure if I will be lucky to survive one more day. Side by side to it, if I will live, will you help me progress the opening of my murder investigation as Marilyn Monroe and bring all the truth out into the light?

Image 130 page 279. Any angel had the right to live. Model. Painter: Dr. Marilyn M. Photographer: Ofer Frohlich

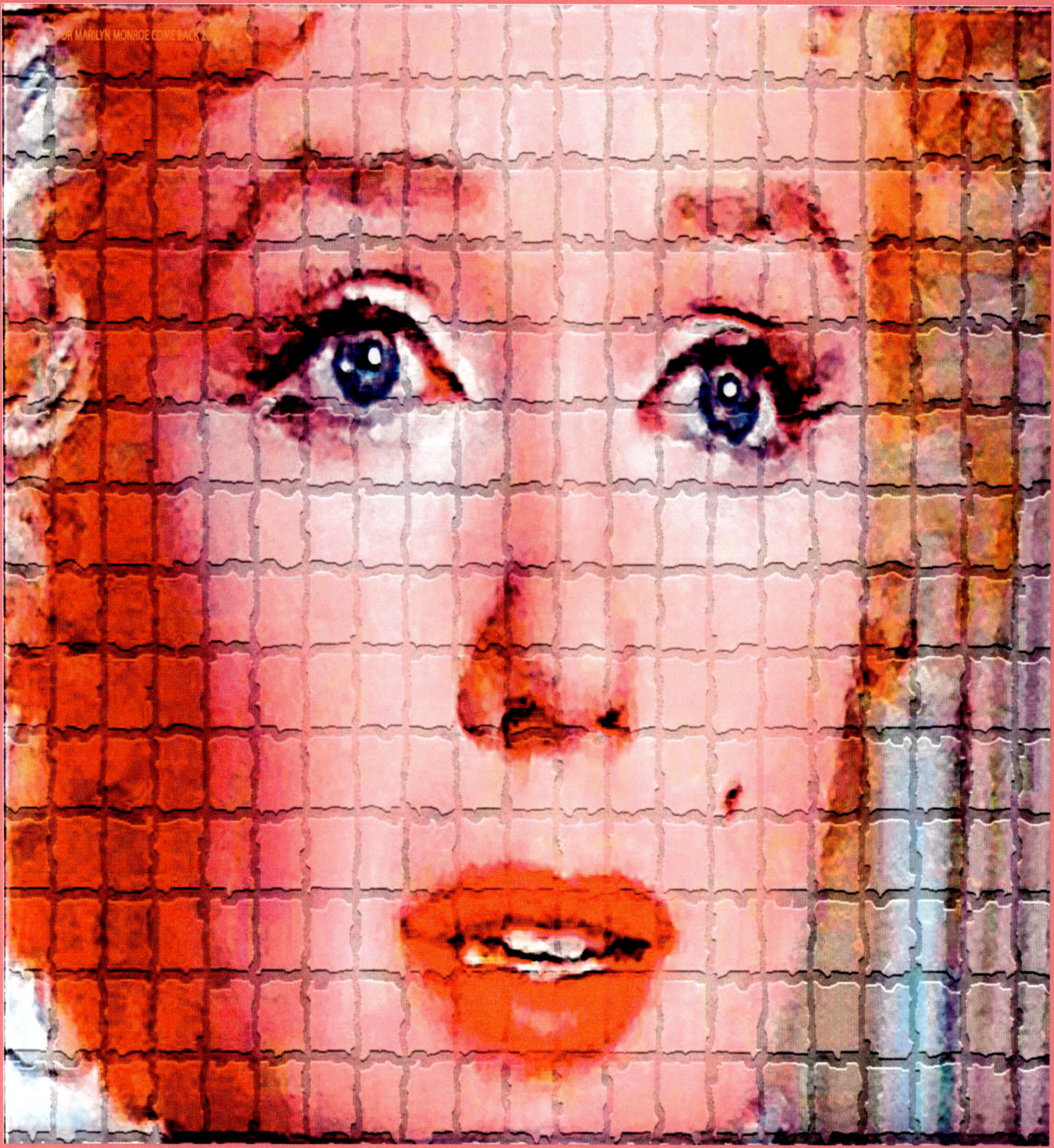
MARILYN MONROE COME BACK

A soul request from Oprah Winfrey

Dear Oprah Winfrey Dr. Bruce Goldberg

was hosted in one of your shows

Dear Oprah Winfrey. Dr. Bruce Goldberg

Who investigated me by hypnosis in my past life

Was hosted in one of your shows

Will you help me progress the opening

Of the investigation around my murder case.

In order to bring all the truth out

Into the light of day

And help bring a full awareness

To the risks all of us women

Are being exposed to

Around the world until today

Image 131 page 281. Any angel had the right to live. Heart. Model. Painter: Dr. Marilyn M. Photographer: Ofer Frohlich

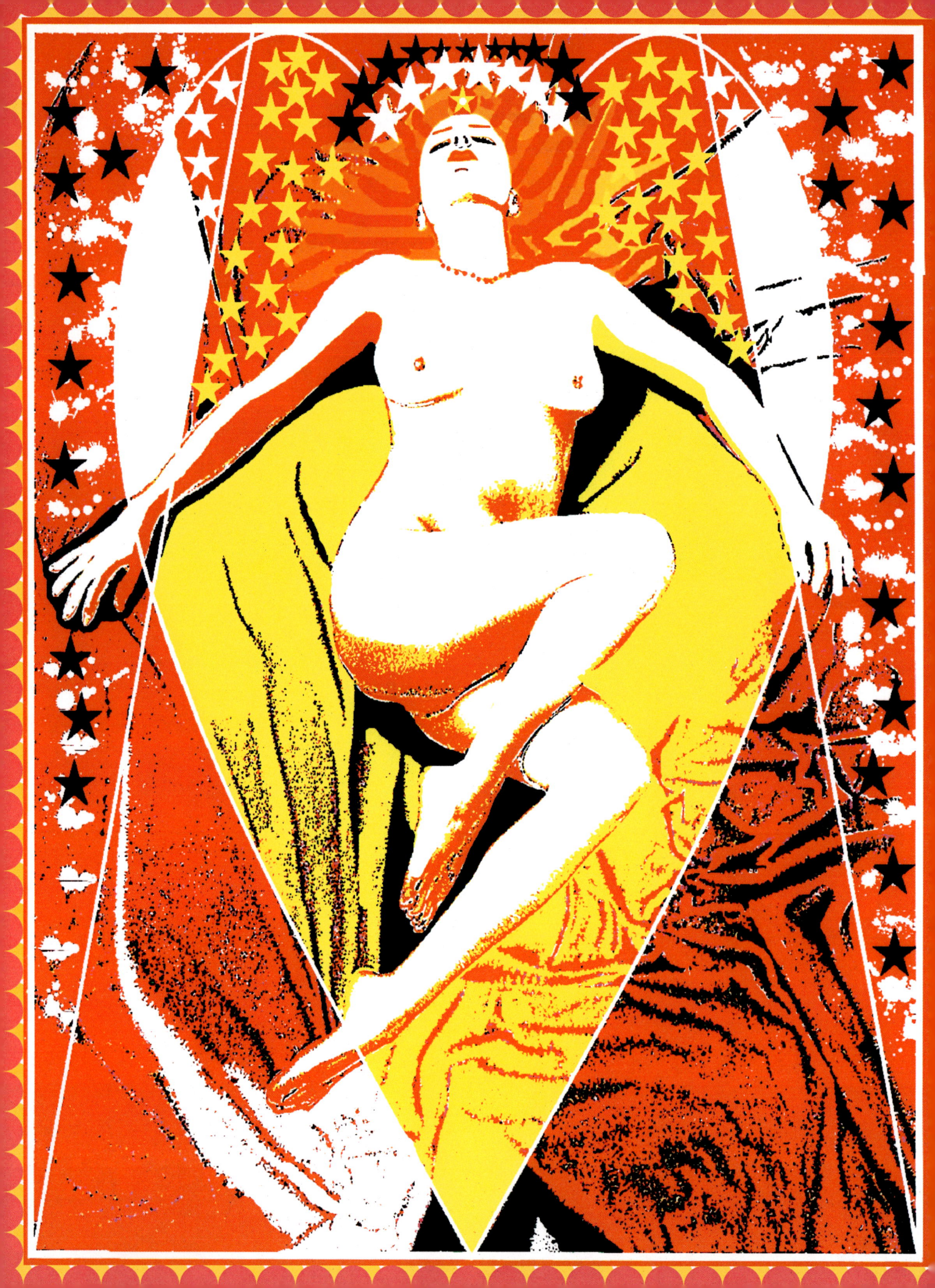

One

The mafia boys

Mr. president. The group of people conducting my death, were from the USA, Japan, and Italy. I am calling this group: The mafia dicks. They celebrated my murder, on my memory death day, by gathering in private parties, sharing stories, secret memories around my execution. The way they Defeated, enslaved, killed the ultimate the queen of all times. It gives them HIGH... SATISFACTION

Few reasons are lying behind my death. They are a universal understanding, behind any women execution around the world from the ancient times until today. It's simple, I become a "headache" for any men, which was conducting my life. As long as I behaved as a sex symbol under their hands everything was ok. From the moment I start to gain power, liberty, freedom, fulfilling all my dreams and desires, with was never in their priorities. I become a "headache". A "pain in their ass". I had to keep making them feel powerful. Wanted. Important. Sexy. With all my natural Golden - Cut essence and different kinds of charms. https://en.wikipedia.org/wiki/Golden_ratio

I felt like I am having many dogs around me, hungry dogs, jingle with their tails, quickly, vigorously. Will you not rub and squeeze them? If I didn't feed them on a steady basis, in one moment they were my best friends, protecting me, the next, they wanted to bite and eat my flesh alive, with their strong teeth. I was a respectable supply of a natural organic health, raw food, of these hungry human dog's beings.

Mr. president. You know how stubborn this special kind of men can be. When they feel they couldn't catch the love they want. They become revengeful. If I wouldn't feed them all day long with my love. Around the clock, I got punished. I had to fill their cup of ego constantly no argue. Everything sets out and become much more complicated, when I started to set my own nest. Hoped to have children.

Image 132 page 283. One. Model. Painter: Dr. Marilyn Monroe. Photographer: Ofer Frohlich

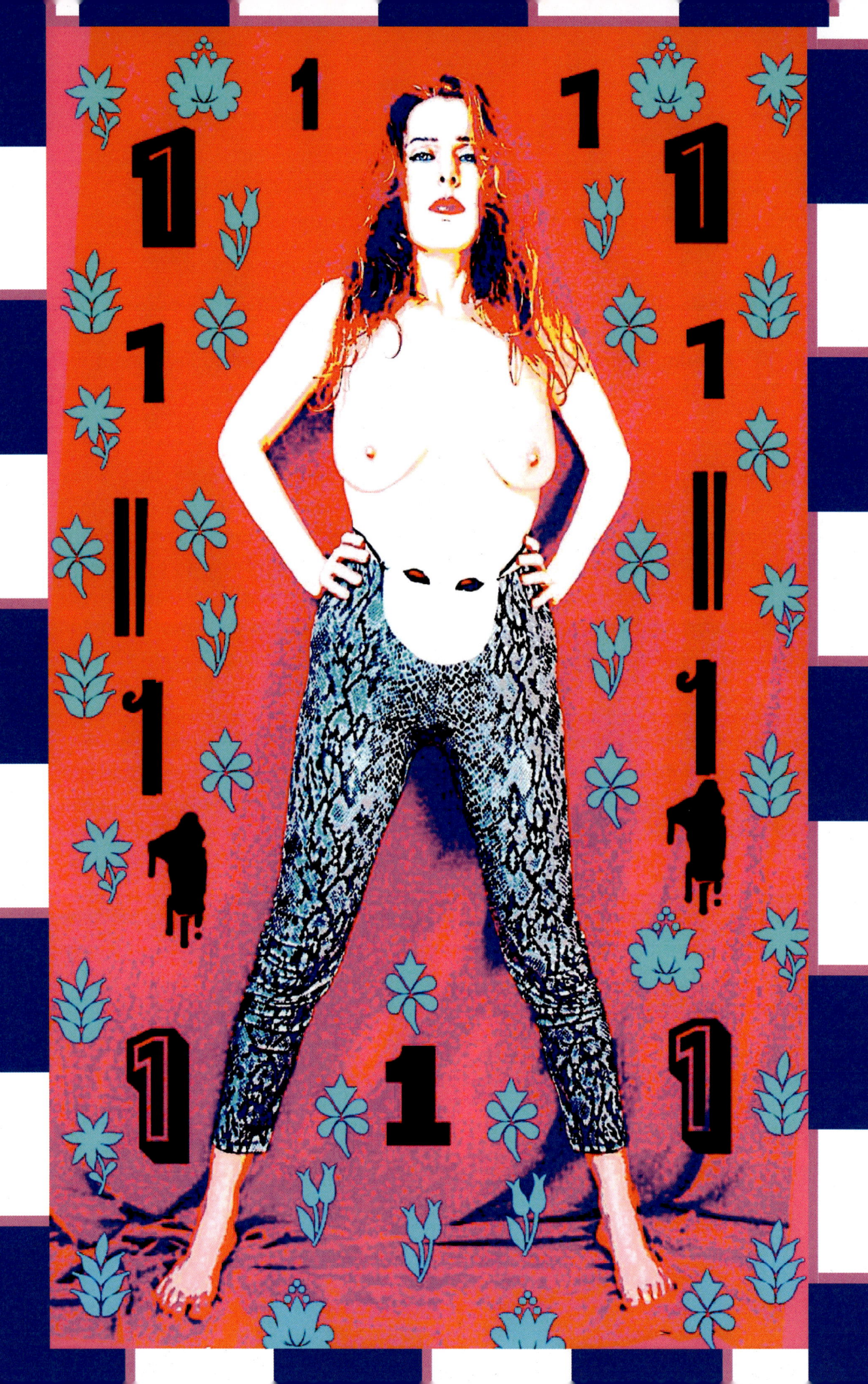

Number One -1 meanings

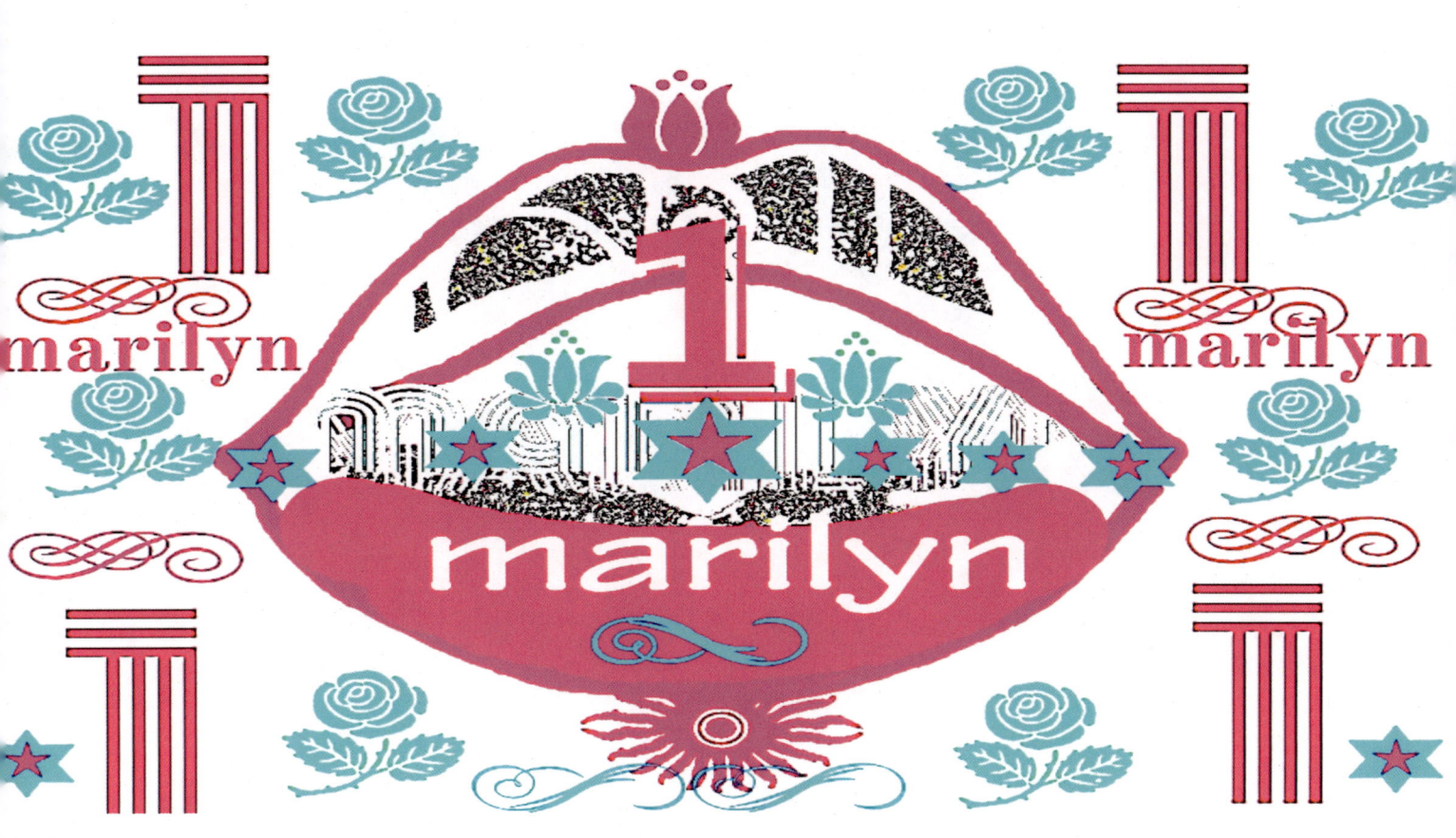

Mercury. Leader, center of the party, determination, self-motivation Accomplishing of goals. Overcome all obstacles, challenge, accomplish supper things, critical of themselves critical of others. Can't tolerate laziness. Independent, need to lead their way Innovation creativity, multitasking, their own boss. Political, military leader. Self-centered. Egotistical, demanding. Arrogant, boastful. Individuality, in love with life, risking it all. Extreme in love with himself

I Want to teach you some special tricks and Magic's

Let me show you boys, What You can do with your eyes closed

When you are touching me real close. Please be tuned. Be polite, not to pee. Not to chirp.

Count with me out aloud until four and then you can break the wall

One…. Two…… Three….. Fourrrrrrrrrrr Yes. That's right, yes yes yes, once more….

Image 133 page 285. Two. Model. Painter: Dr. Marilyn Monroe. Photograph: Ofer Frohlich

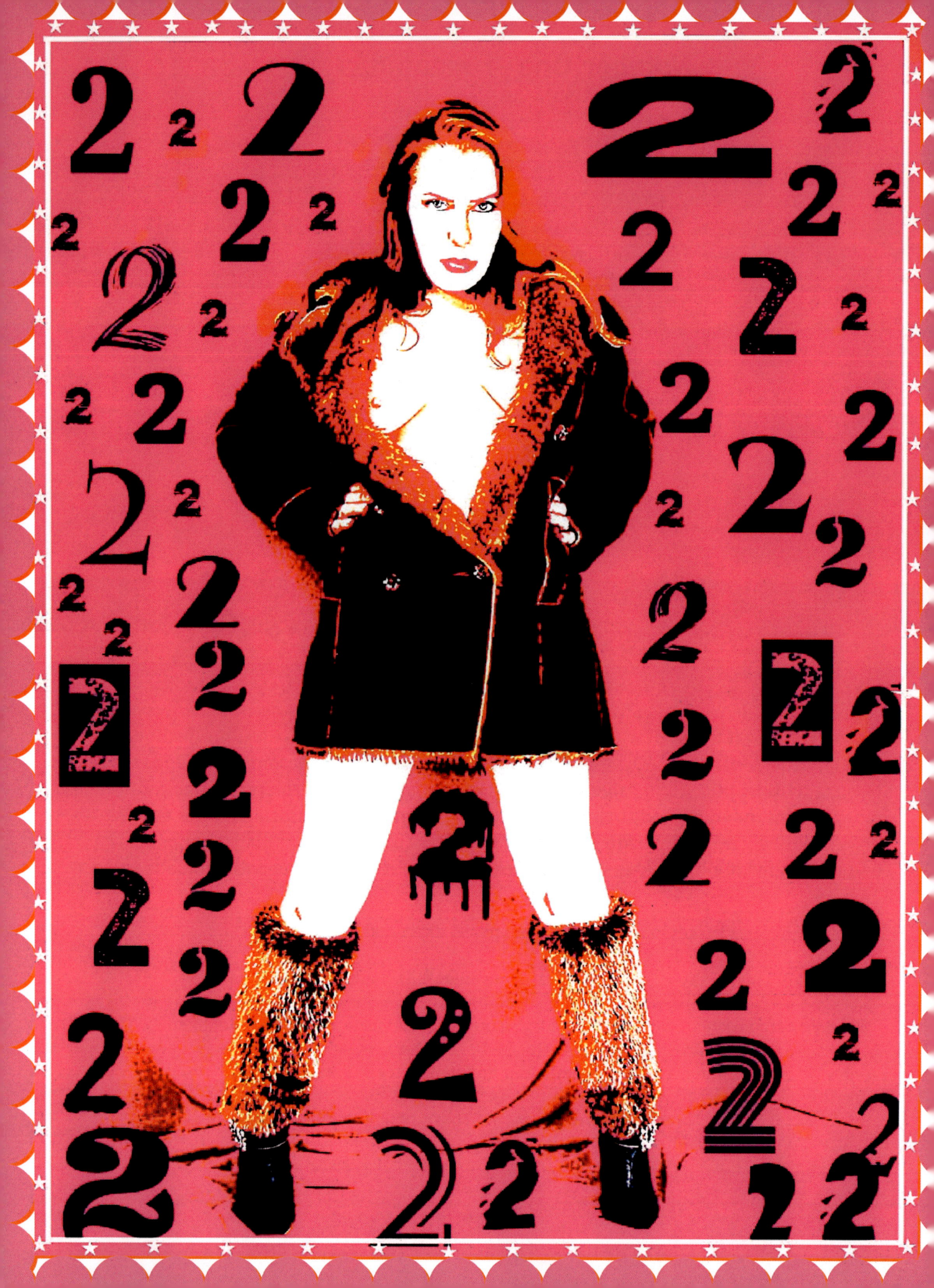

Two

Baby girl or boy

Mr. president. When I own my own company, my attitude changed a little. I began to put myself before others. From the no condition attitude everyone becomes accustomed to it. I begin to define boundaries. Especially each time, when I got into pregnancy. Only, men, felt with their unnatural ability to smell a woman, by her hormones, I am pregnant. Immediately, each time when I got pregnant, at the first month, they start to crawl over and around me like a group of snakes, crawling into the bird nest to steal her eggs. They felt my baby's by their animal, human instinct, knowing they are going to steal my mother's attention from them. They felt extreme jealousy toward any natural never been born baby's. Fear they will take their place.

My baby life had been under a great danger and a risk, even before they been born. No wonder, I gave so many natural abortions. I instinctively felt it, my womb as well, immediately reacted to it. My nest was not protected from all the wolf around. Then my womb, faced a natural miscarriage. Just before some damage will harm my baby's. My womb had delivered them before their time, as a self-protection action, make my baby's run away from me, as if knowing, my womb is not a safe place to grow up inside of. It happened always between the 1-9 weeks of pregnancy. I felt an internal bewitched, hex, spelled. It was like watching a car accident happening to me, and keeps running inside of me over and over again, I watched how my babies are running away from my open womb, while these snake men, were waiting for them, devour them alive as they went out.

Not once in my pregnancies, I could not run according to all prospects. Impregnated by a most known married president, this baby was the public foe, even before they spoil their first month of conception, my little child caught inside of the wires of a dangerous love. I felt I could not protect them. I knew, becoming the John. F. Kennedy, wife instead of Jackie, will immediately make of me the public enemy. Only I was so in love, both with john and God. Each time when John touched me, I felt I was in paradise, as if god is touching me, penetrating me, with his fire, and light.

It was a mystical moment for me, to be with John, a spiritual moment, not a physical one as each of you sees it. I felt John is part of my soul, of my blood and core, we were alike, two sides of the same coin. When his eyes were looking at me, while he was inside of me, my breath was knocked out of my chest, looking deeply into his eyes, I could witness Jesus is looking back at me. Basically, Jackie got her France army. I didn't produce so many Jewish fans as she performed with her France army. I was extremely naïve, I didn't realize, John, besides making love with me, sees in me, a dangerous woman for his family, which can bring on his: Reputation. Marriage a complete disaster and catastrophe. One side of him had fun with me, the other was on guard.

Number Two - 2 meanings

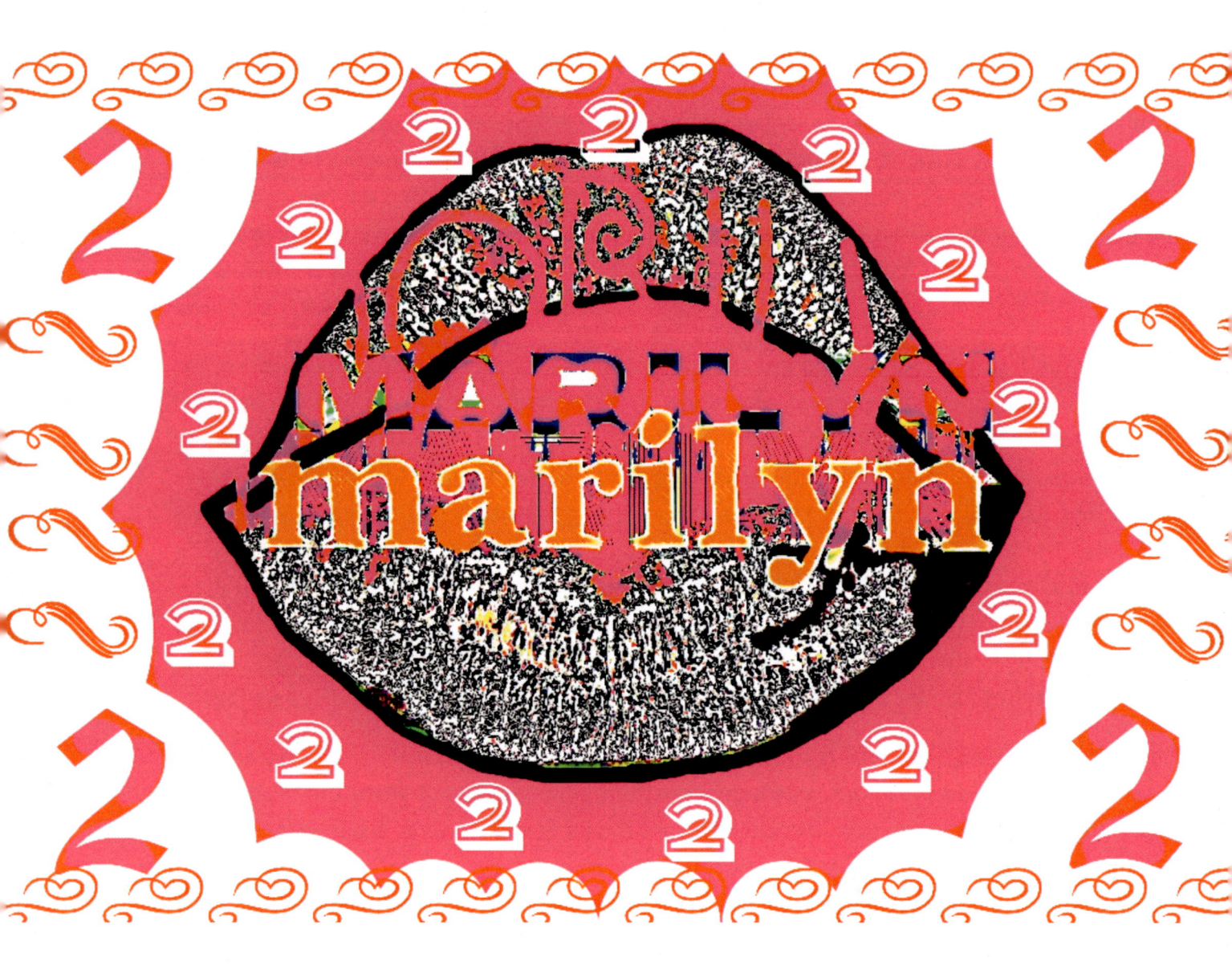

Venus. Feminine, very underestimated, very diplomatic, forgiving understanding. A Peacemaker avoids confrontations, ultimate survivor. Under attack flexible, then strike back, like a snake tongue split in two, bending backward before striking, the power behind the throne. The kind wife, cunning, relies on the advice of allies. Grace, sensuality, flattering attentive psychologist. Sophistication, the sense of music, rhythm, a dancer, sense of humor, witty Cut her contractors to pieces. Emotional, demanding, expects to be treated as a princess Devoted, expects devotion. A drama queen, need of attention, not materialistic at all. Much graceful.

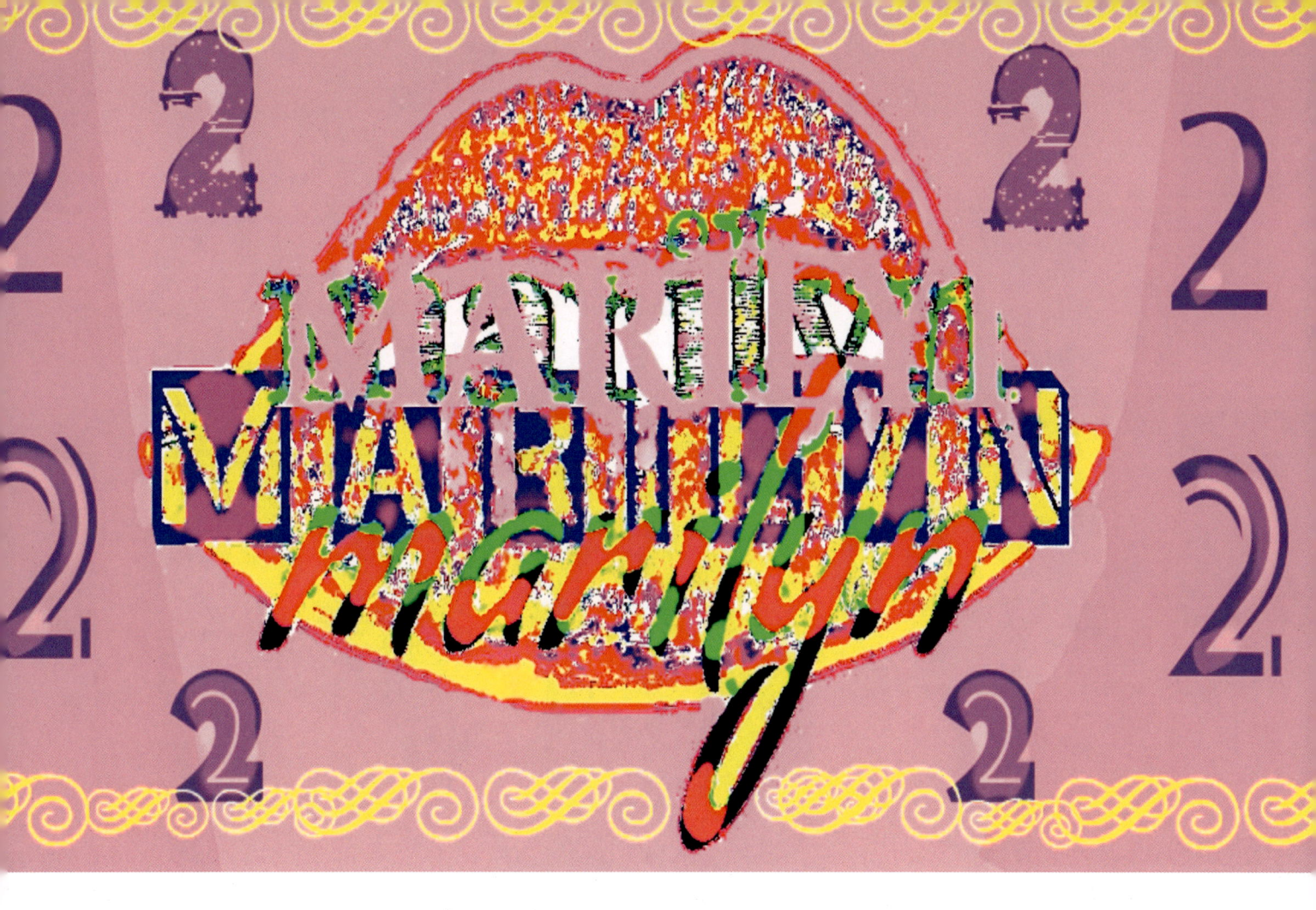

Two crazy diamonds we are, dancing on a floor

Two sides of a golden king coin

Hovering with passion, melted inside one another

Dancing naked to the melodic beats hearts

Flying high like no bird could fly up above the sky

A gentle wind from heaven pulling oxygen into our lungs

Two crazy diamonds dancing to the godly rhythm of passion

Covered with the vibration of the universal music

Do. Re. Mi. Fa. Sol. La. Si. Do. Do. Si. La. Sol. Fa. Mi. Re. Do

Image 134 page 289. Three. Model. Painter: Dr. Marilyn Monroe. Photographer: Ofer Frohlich

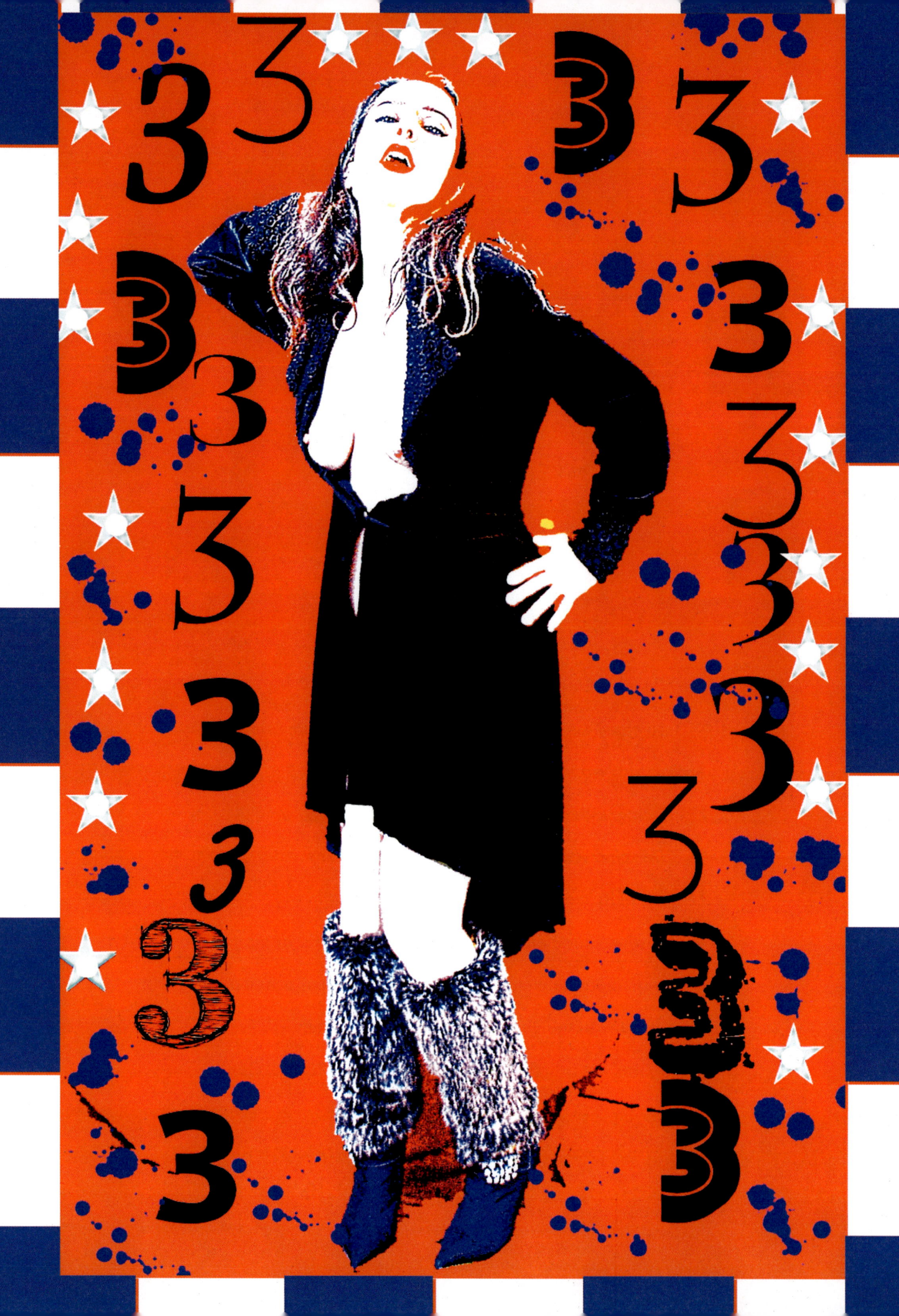

Three

Jacqueline. Where are my baby's

Mr. president. I am not pointing away; John was the one which executed me. He was and will always be my soul mate. Unfortunately, he needed to choose between me, and his wife Jackie. She'd won. Her eggs won. I genuinely looked up to her, she was a courageous woman, firm women, she got this instinct of an iron woman, not as did. She knew all about keeping boundaries. She knew, not as I didn't, to keep them firmly, gently with a smile. She knew to keep a man in his Testicles. Something any woman needs to learn to do, if she is experiencing a stable house, she needs to go on, she needs to know, how to keep her man. If she is sustaining a stable father, which adores her, as the most precious baby girl, he has got in the whole world, it is a lot more comfortable for her, to hold back what belongs to her, to herself. I didn't get this kind of attitude, of a stable home, or a father.

I got other powers, people called all these powers, under the rubric of "a sex symbol". This is pathetic, since I have got so much more than this. At some point of time, Jackie, had started to copy my voice, my look, the way I move, and all other kinds of characters. She already caught, so much then I could place my hands on: John my soul mate, was belonged to her. His children, the president of USA wife title, her special style. She was a very good looking, all she needed was to add to it my voice. In order to become more perfect.

Thanks god, she didn't dive her hair to blond, or made some nude photos in the pool as I did, and that's it, she could own as well my sex symbol title. Thanks god she was not brave enough, and her place in that frame of time, didn't allow her to bend against the tuning she needed to be, to the public opinion. She could never cross all the line as I could. So, at last, I left with something, not for a long time. It was just a matter of time, until they will take it all away from me. I was listed, at the black list, to be fully executed.
https://en.wikipedia.org/wiki/Jacqueline_Kennedy_Onassis

My poor John, he needed to make a devastating decision. Choosing between his wife and me, between my babies, made of pure passion, love and lust, and Jackie. Both were the fruit of his passionate, wisdom and love. If the world were more open at that time, John could have Jackie baby's, as well mine. Choosing between me and Jackie, was like choosing between his natural soul which I represent, to his platform profile made by the public, which Jackie represented. This unnatural formal image of himself, was finally forced on him. The public, the government, Jackie army, won. They made of him my enemy. But, inside of his heart, nothing was different, this was driving me crazy, I didn't realize he is not powerful as I thought, to inflict his will on the world. Our babies could bring so much wisdom, to the world. https://en.wikipedia.org/wiki/John_F._Kennedy

Number Three - 3 meanings

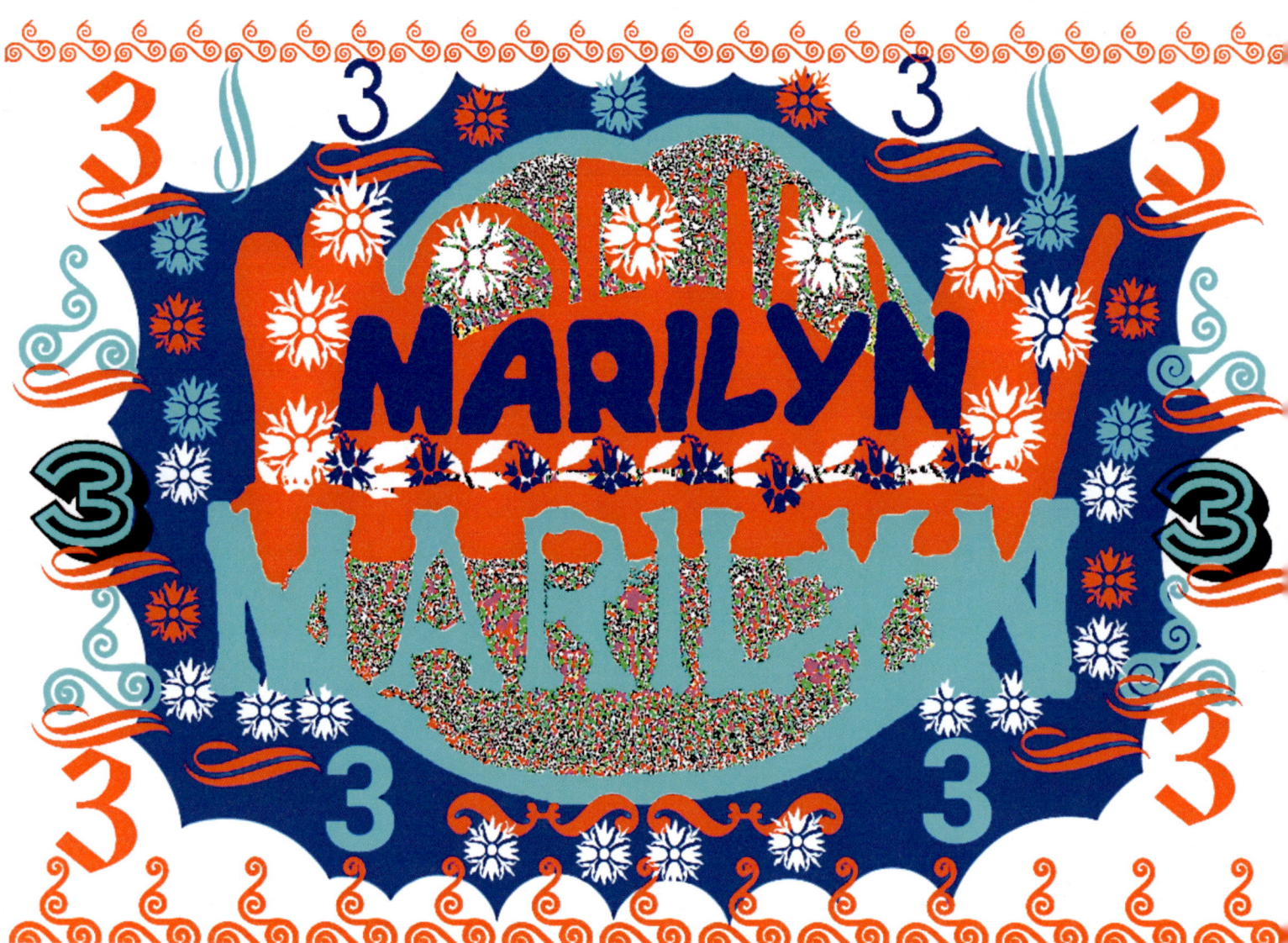

Earth. Optimism, shuns, joy, inspiration, creativity, communication Imagination, intelligence sociability, society, friendliness, kindness, compassion. Humor, energy expansion increase spontaneity, synthesis, heaven-human-hell, past-present-future thought Feeling-action comprehensive, Optimistic, fun-loving, a 'joker', the charismatic. Enlivening, youthful, elegant, jumping, funny, enthusiastic. Idealistic, fulfillment, encouragement, assistance, skills, culture, pleasure Freedom, adventure, exuberance, brave, rhythm, a master, divine, peace, clarity, love within, Indifference, concentration, spectacular, mood swings, performing arts fruitfulness Happiness, creator, entertaining, social. Keen, luxurious, expansion, against routines, star Venus, attractive, dynamic, extrovert, arrogant, exhibitionist.

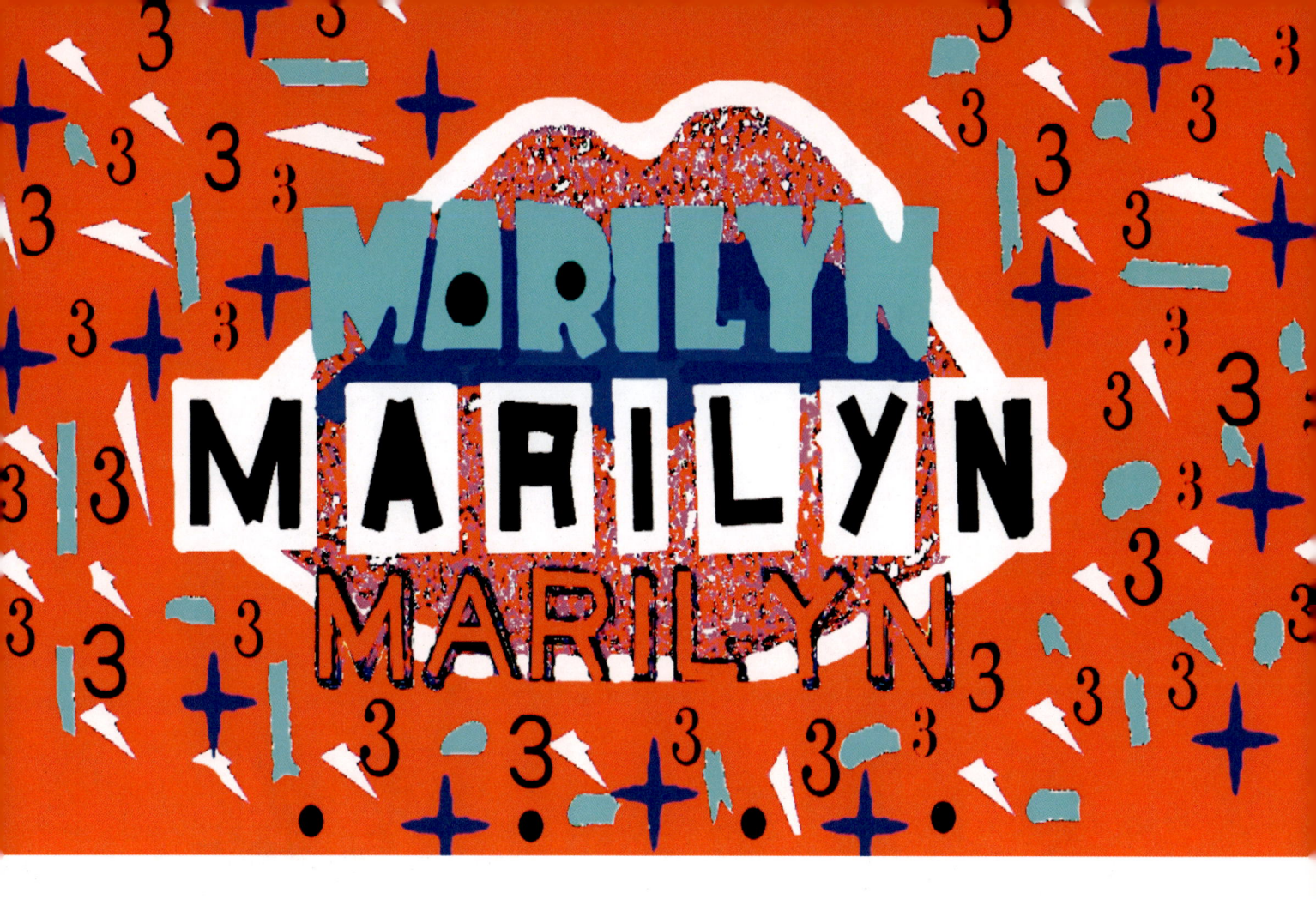

Jacky, she is, a little kid, I am playing with the kindergarten

She is pushing me, taking my dolls

I told her to stop. Move away, stop pushing

Stop tearing my hair

Stop cutting my doll, Give me her scissors.

Stop pushing so hard

Stop using her knight.

Noooooo Jacky… Noooooooooooo

Please stopppppp.

Image 135 page 293. Four. Model. Painter: Dr. Marilyn Monroe. Photographer: Ofer Frohlich

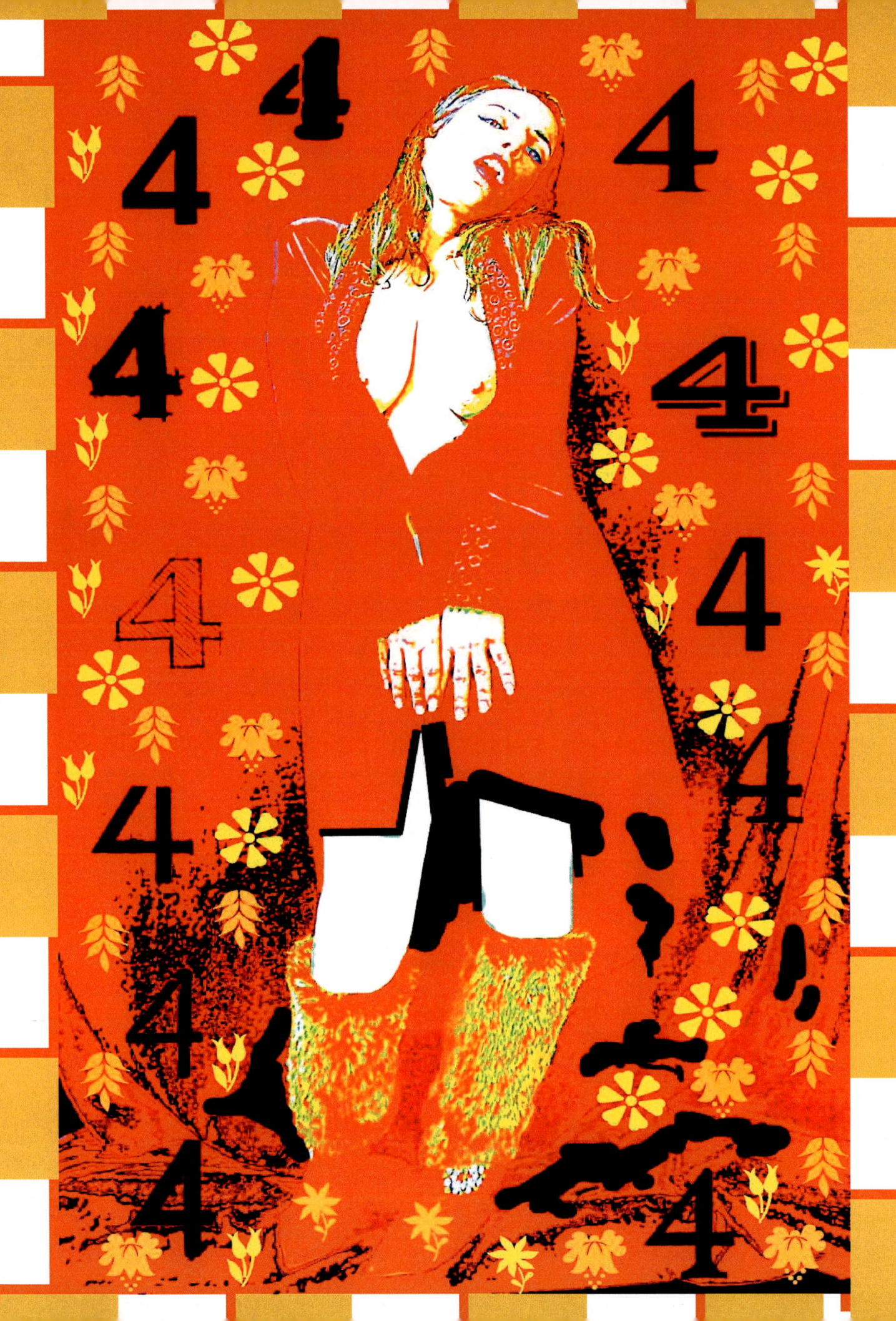

Four

The Art of Killing Marilyn continues ver 1

Mr. President. Everybody hopes to share pieces of me, own parts, used parts, people feel stronger while using me like using a drug, I help them be, full with self-energy, self-love, and self-esteem, self-importance, self-confident, cheerful and optimistic. My executors understood this side effect I produced, the same as a drug do. The ability to influence people all around the globe with my smile. I mentioned earlier, they used an actress, looks alike me. In order to perform my living shape, inside of my home, instead of my dead body, she was executed, and performed the look alike me inside of my funeral. The mafia boys knew, my precious body, should not be wasted for the interest of the worms. The executors knew the monetary value; they can obtain from my body.

My funeral was merely an exhibition, in front of the public eyes. The look alike me was buried instead of me in my tomb. They put her on my makeup, dressed her with my dress. At the same time, my original organs were set up to sell, as an exceptional piece of Marilyn artwork, inside of a big auction. The tissues around my organs, were meant to give their last perform at "the last feast with Marilyn", served as a special delicious dinner, contain my soft internal delicious body parts. One particular human was responsible for my body. He revealed to me, while grooming me for the rituals ahead, how he is going to prepare my body parts, for this last supper dish. I was laughing. Thinking he is telling me a jock. It was the side effect, of the laughter drugs that was pooled inside of me, together with the finest red wine, to make me cooperative in my last hours.

This special human, was called: "The Duke". Responsible for keeping my body refresh, beautiful. Particular after my death, revealed to me the methods, with it, he will employ after I will pass away. How he will slay all the worms inside of my interior organs, will wash my parts carefully, prepare them for the auction and the dish. He continues too pure his story around me, how some percentage parts are going to be sold, as a rare art piece, others as a food. The remainder of my external body will be exhibiting as a mummy, he said. This outside shell of me, will be held as a unique sculpture, presenting at an underground exhibition, on my eternal name. Marilyn forever. Just before I will be dead, he said, at the auction itself. I delivered to perform myself on a particular stage in nude. I was used to perform in nude, thinking he is talking an artistic nonsense. They need to see the item before they buy it, he said, there for above the stage, they will place a big TV screen, together with a mirror, reflecting me from all directions along the auction, as one piece. Then, I will be exhibiting once more, after death, with all my internal organs, my organs will be exhibiting on a special illustration of a big diamond, of 100000 carats.

Image 136 page 295. Four. Model. Painter: Dr. Marilyn Monroe. Photographer: Ofer Frohlich

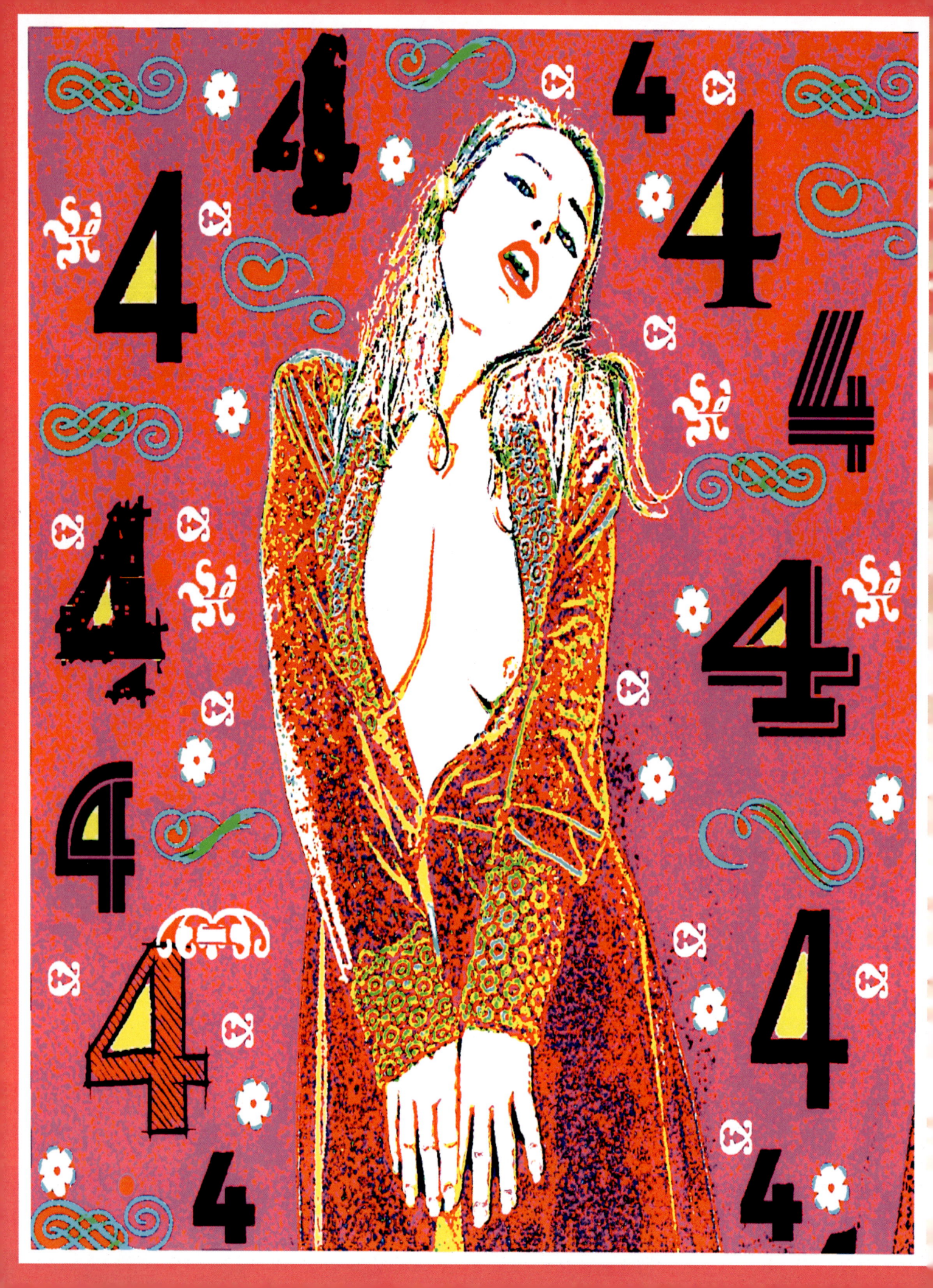

Number Four – 4 meanings

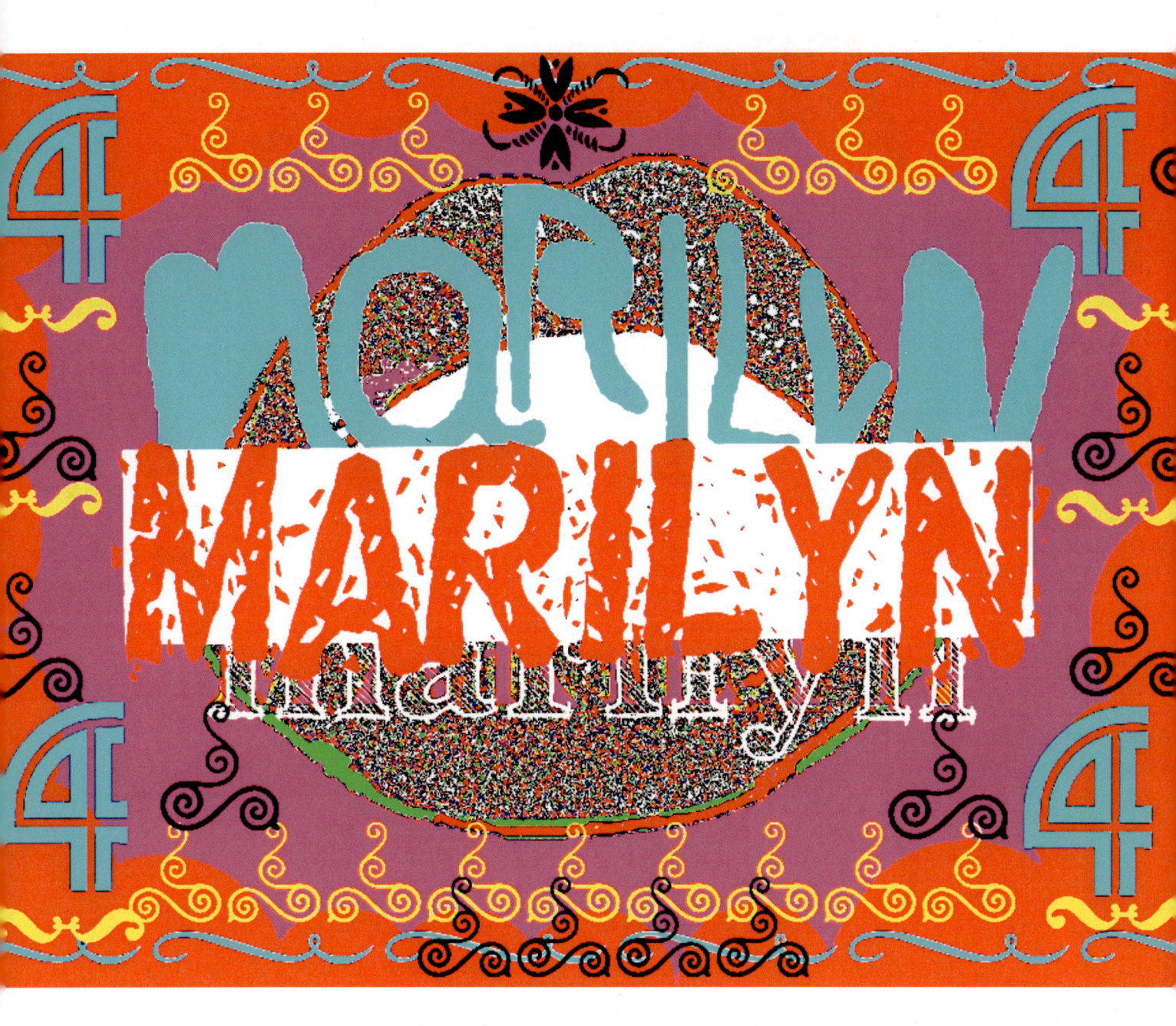

Mars. terminal, practical, down-to-earth, expectation of others Organized, proper place Sense of right and wrong, honest, Loyal, dependable, physically healthy Strong, neat, clean no attention desire, fight for territory. Goal-oriented, excellent memory Workaholic, neither creative nor artistic, a good provider, demands discipline, loyalty, panic attacks. Needs things fully under control. Excellent friend, partner, stubborn, rigid, serious. Truth teller. Cautious, miss opportunities, very grounded, analytical, very disciplined. Like routine. Like to be at home. Like bed.

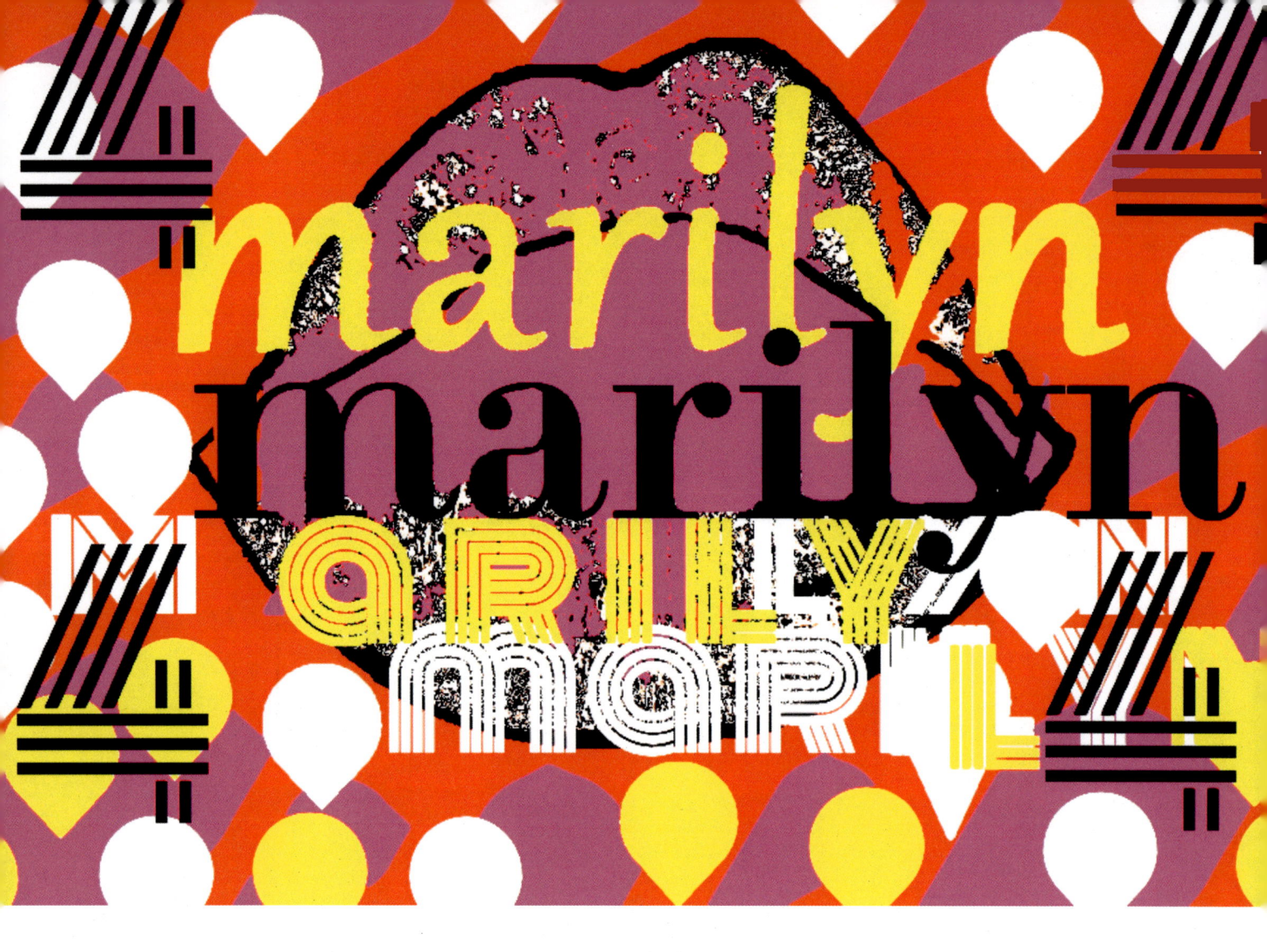

Their eyes were like a giant spider crawling around my body searching for nourishment

Trying to get inside my flesh, into my soft parts waiting to give a bite in my bare skin

I tried to disappear inside of my own womb, try to bring out this ancient shadow

Onto the surface of my skin. Clean the pain and release my soul from their trance

Protect me from the spider wolves eating my bones. God. Help me wear out the crush

of stone around me. Put a white flag in the middle of the red war

Fading diffusing into the unknown. My ray of sunlight needs to break into the blue sky

Go back home, let my soul be grounded. Like the number four.

Five

Marilyn organs

Mr. president. Do you know, what was the value of each of my organs back in, 1962, and what are their values today? I could be so rich today, if I could have just 1% of my value today. Instead, I am very poor, while everyone gets richer by me. Is always the shoemaker going barefoot? Can you imagine me in my past life, instead of being a sex symbol, what would be my life looks like, If I was a shoemaker? Then, I could have much more money. I could earn money by selling a polished shoe, be alive, and have children. My family in this present got a shoe store, I am not kidding, I know to sell shoes, I could be a great shoes seller. I could be a millionaire owning many shoe stores around the globe. Should I jump back in time into my past life, choose a different path? Instead of a " sex symbol", a" living legend sexy shoe stocker". I could be today 89 and still shell shoes.

Instead, what I have got: I am dead, with no shoes to cover my bare feet. With no $ in my bank. Since I have, such a big trauma from the power of earning money and fame, I can't let myself be more than a very poor woman. I don't want to be murdered again. My sub conscience keeps me alive with 0 $ in my bank. But let not spoil, to the animal humans their appetite, let see, how my organs were exhibited, finally bravely sold, at my last auction let watch the list of organs for sale: Marilyn heart. Marilyn Kidneys. Marilyn Spain. Marilyn Colony. Marilyn Brain. Marilyn Liver. Marilyn Lungs. Even my vocal cords were sold for the best price. My Spain. My Uterus. I believe as well my last ovum. Who knows, I may have one child or even more around the world, I don't know of Impregnation with my last mature ovum. I wonder who is the father. Maybe, the one who paid the best price for my other sex videos, I hope he has gotten some good genes. As I did. Mr. president. I lived my life like a butterfly, with beautiful colors on my wings, without knowing, my wings will be burnt. I was defined, my beauty can change the cruel man's soul. I spoil them with my charm make of them a good boy. I didn't have a realization; they are a mafia of devil boys.

As in any mafia, these men were practiced to produce, whatever they want with a blink. They could not stand up to see, how easy it was for other men, to catch with me into bed, while they can't render me into their layer as they wanted, it didn't yield them any satisfaction, to hear about one more love story I took toward the word. To see me happy in the arms of another man, was a torment for them, full with jealousy. This internal dissatisfaction, was like a hidden atomic bomb. It made them break the conspiracy secrecy elimination contract with me, in order to accept a full command over me, take everything they demanded for themselves. My body, mind, and soul.

Image 137 page 299. Five. Model. Painter: Dr. Marilyn Monroe. Photographer: Ofer Frohlich

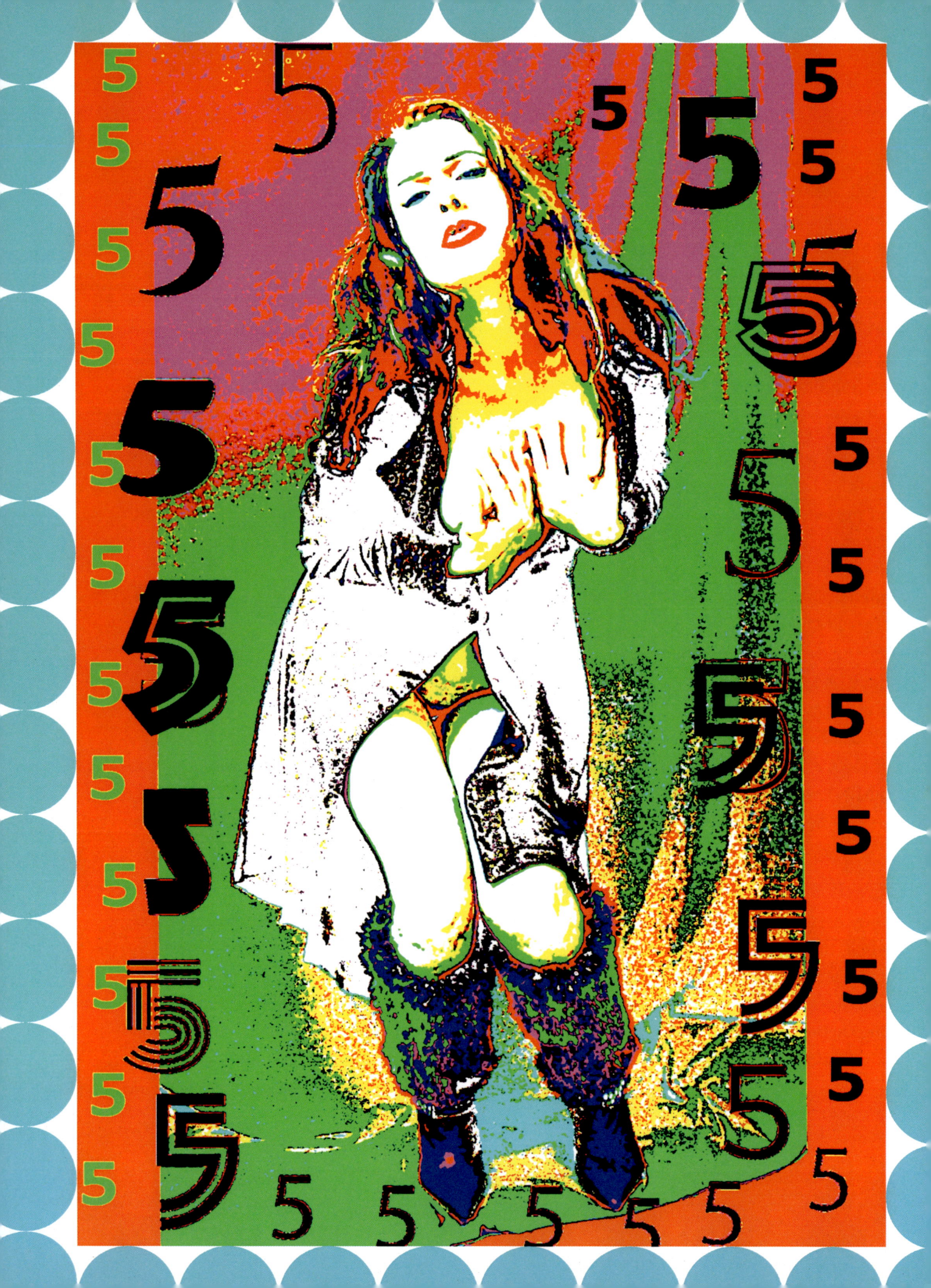

Number Five – 5 meanings

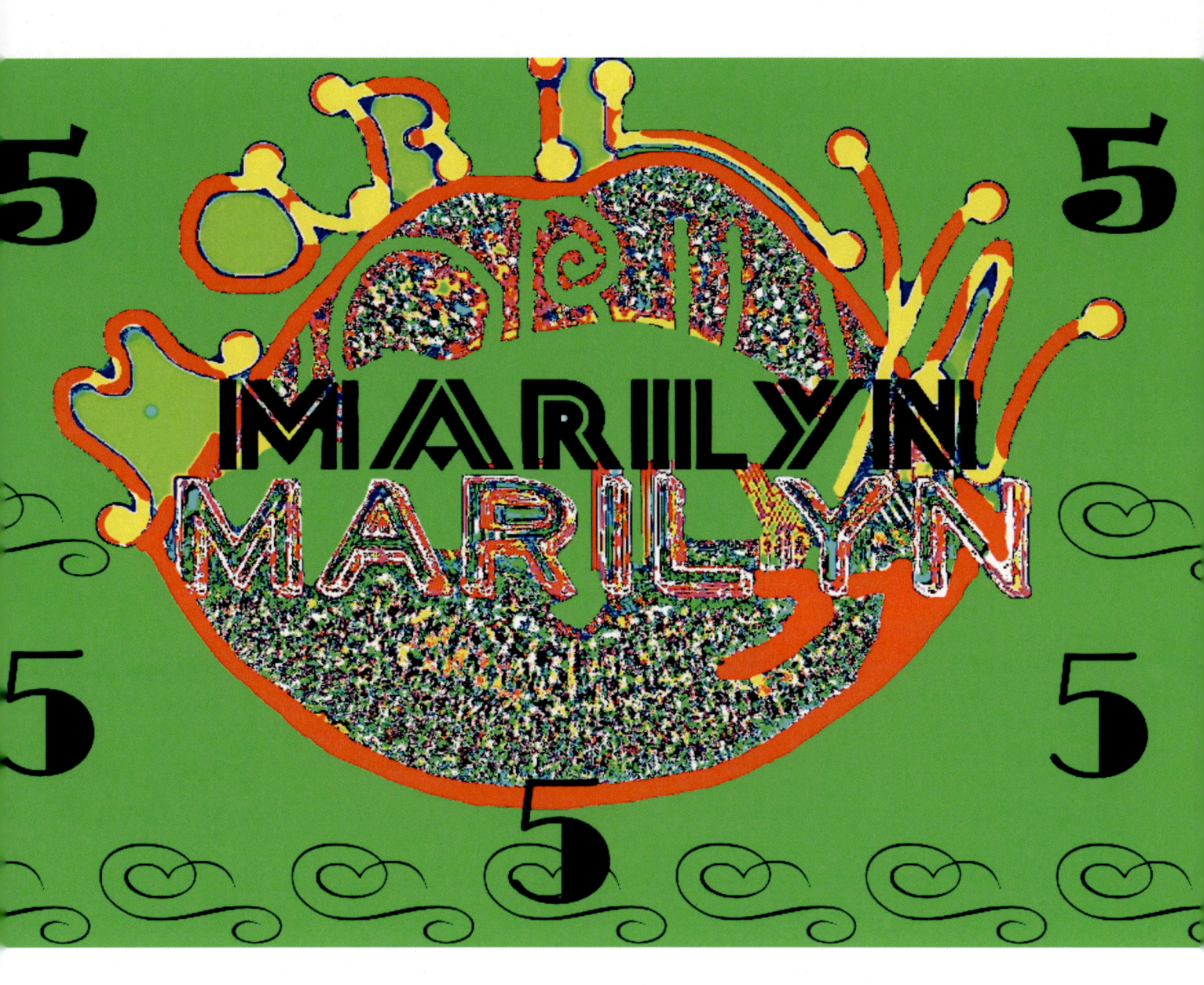

Jupiter. James Monroe, fifth president of the USA fight against slavery Protection against the evil eye. Hamsa – five it the flame of Miriam - the sister of Moses. 5 books of the Torah. Luther Rose. David the king killed Goliath with five pebbles. Freedom. Rebels against dogmas, ideologies, adventurous, daredevil nature, so flexible, converted, healthy sense of humor Selfish, thoughtless, not considers the future, not worrying. Procrastinate experiment with sex, drugs, alcohol. Lack of discipline, restraint, dynamic motion. Random. Like to run, jump. Fly ride on horses.

I had Immune myself from the mafia boy's.

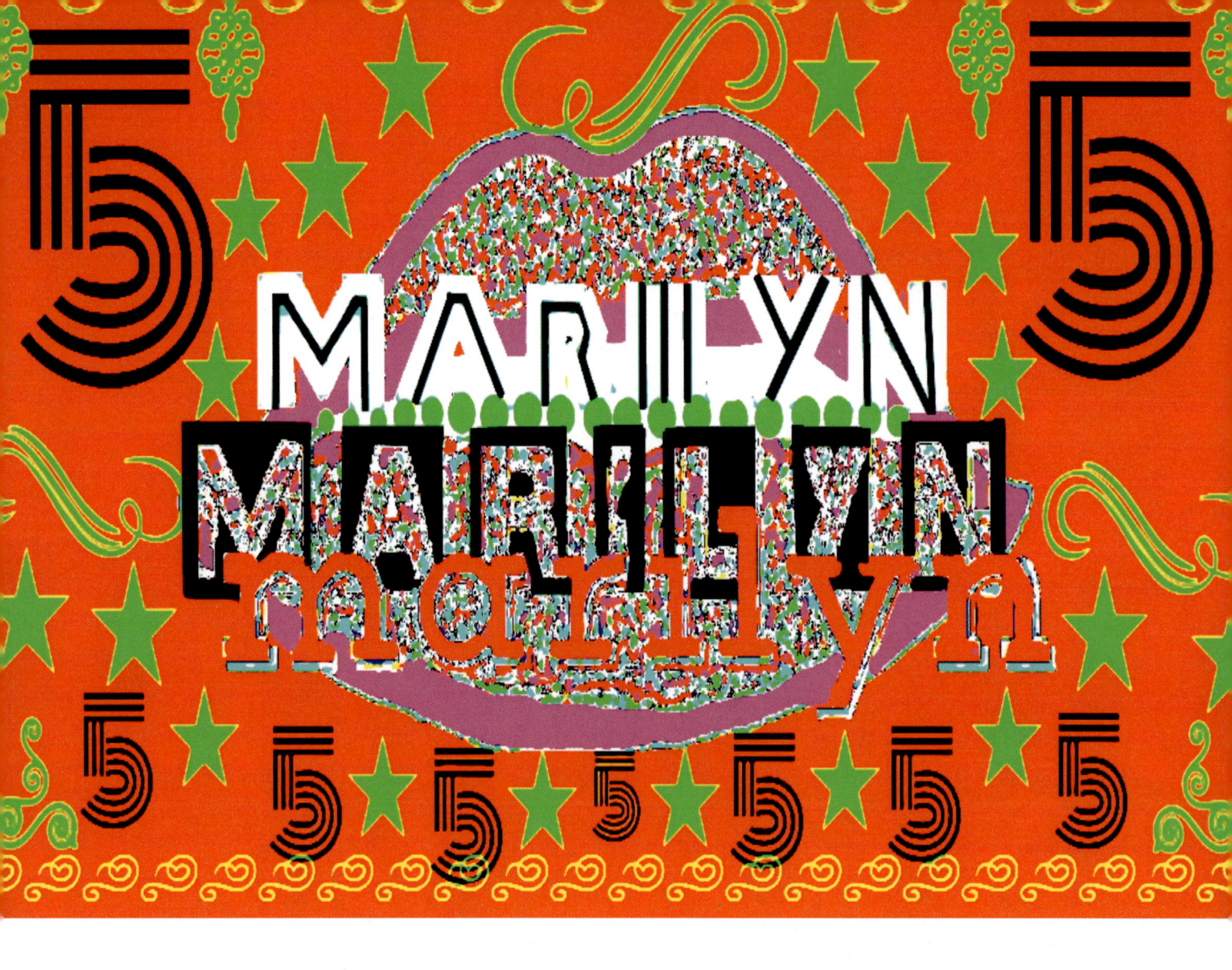

These energetic life sucker's bacteria

Squeezing people, choking Dreams

I am not your slave, or doll, I am a liberal soul

Bursting out from your electric walls

Hiding in a place you will never find me

Trusting in God, he will protect me

From your selfish crocodile brain

Six

The beauty and the beast

Mr. President. Most of my life I felt as an ox inside of a stadium, in front of the Red Velvet. This is the main symbol which accompanying me. From the past on the Red Velvet made with Tom Kelley Sr. Into the present. Taurus, an ox, is my zodiac luck in both lives. The Red Velvet provokes around me a military activity, this color runs after me all the way from my past, to remain me, of my drops of my soul mixed with the drops of blood, crying from the Center of the earth to set free. http://en.wikipedia.org/wiki/Red. The red color, stands for beautiful things as: roses. Dedication. The mythical goddess of love, Aphrodite. The mythical goddess of the Greek and Roman - Venus. The cross bloodshed Christianity. The Jewish painted their doors with their red blood, during the plague of the firstborn for protection. Red is the traditional color of the Virgin Mary, the color wears a Santa Claus. At the Beauty and the Beast, a film made in 1991, the main symbol along the cinema is the ruby rose. http://en.wikipedia.org/wiki/Beauty_and_the_Beast_(1991_film)

The beauty and the beast cycle of life, had continued to be a living part inside of me. Men act toward me as the beast. I as a woman was the beauty. The public enjoys to recognize with the beauty, they didn't want to recognize the beast hovering about me, let not forget, the overall humanity is afraid of dying from the beast. The animal side which was resonant inside of me, was a reflection of my mother, Gladys, rapist, my unknown father. All the human beings around me, could not stand, my father wildness parts, hiding inside of me. They have to kill me, to kill his seeds inside of me. Mr. president. Are you still with me? Are you awake or asleep? Can You see the mathematician? When I was 19 years old at the present, I painted a couple of hugging horses. Beauty white angelic horses, represents the female, next to it, a red horse with a face of a wolf beast represents the men. The original painting was stolen from me from my bedroom. Right after my mother, Sarah passed away. Somebody close to the family or in it, had stolen it.

Joe DiMaggio, and Arthur Miller, my husbands, wanted to protect me, from the sexuality I shared with the public, which was about to end my life, and they felt it. For men, can feel the danger around a woman. Which other men reflect, recognize other men hiding motivation, which I didn't. They felt they cannot protect me from other adult males, plus a big pressure on them, from the mafia, threatened their lives, forced them to divorce me or they will be dead. This manipulative attitude, done, in order to have a free access to me. The mafia boss, had to get rid of my husband, each time I got one.

Image 138 page 303. Six. Model. Painter: Dr. Marilyn Monroe. Photographer: Ofer Frohlich

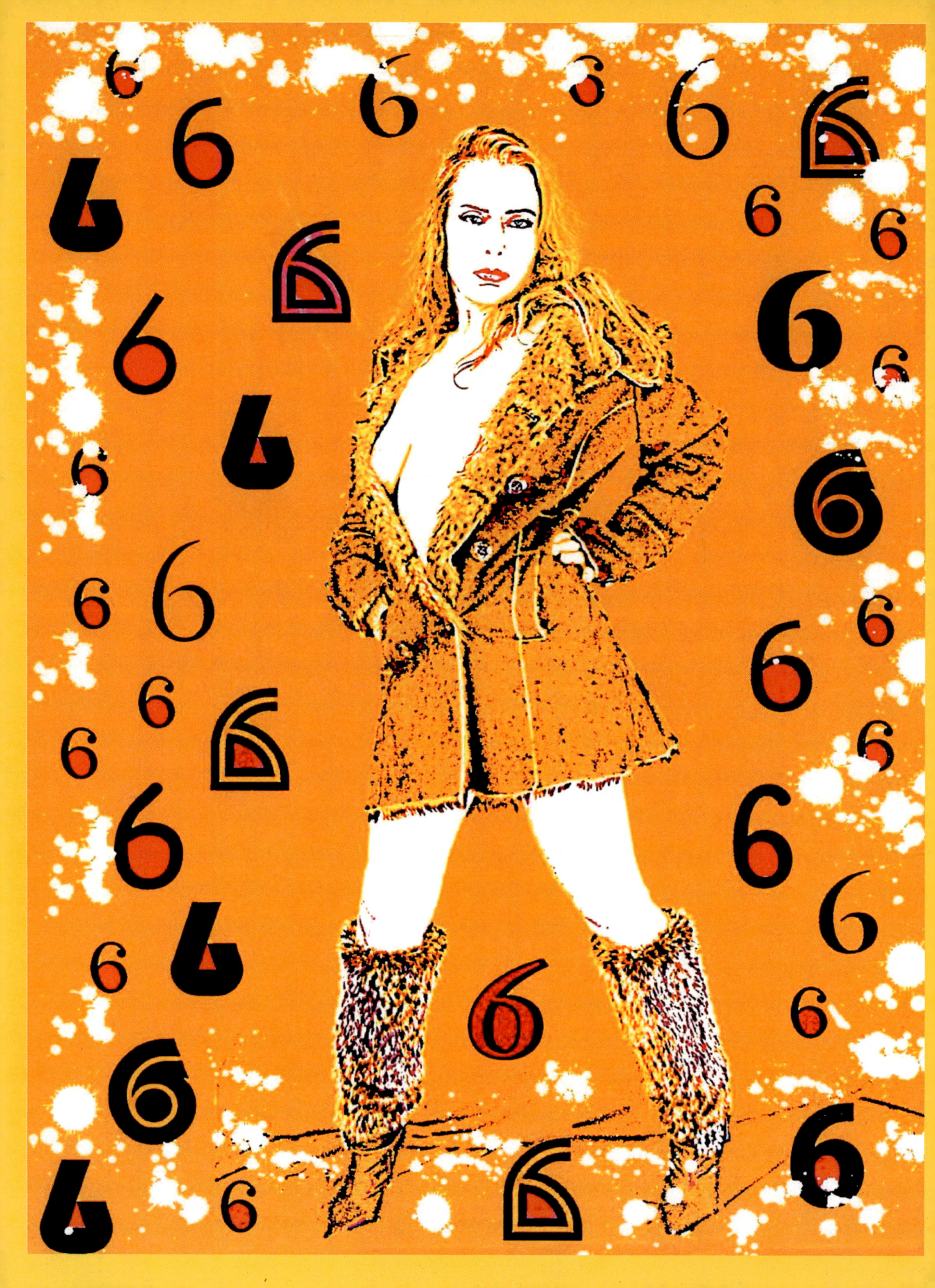

Number Six - 6 meanings

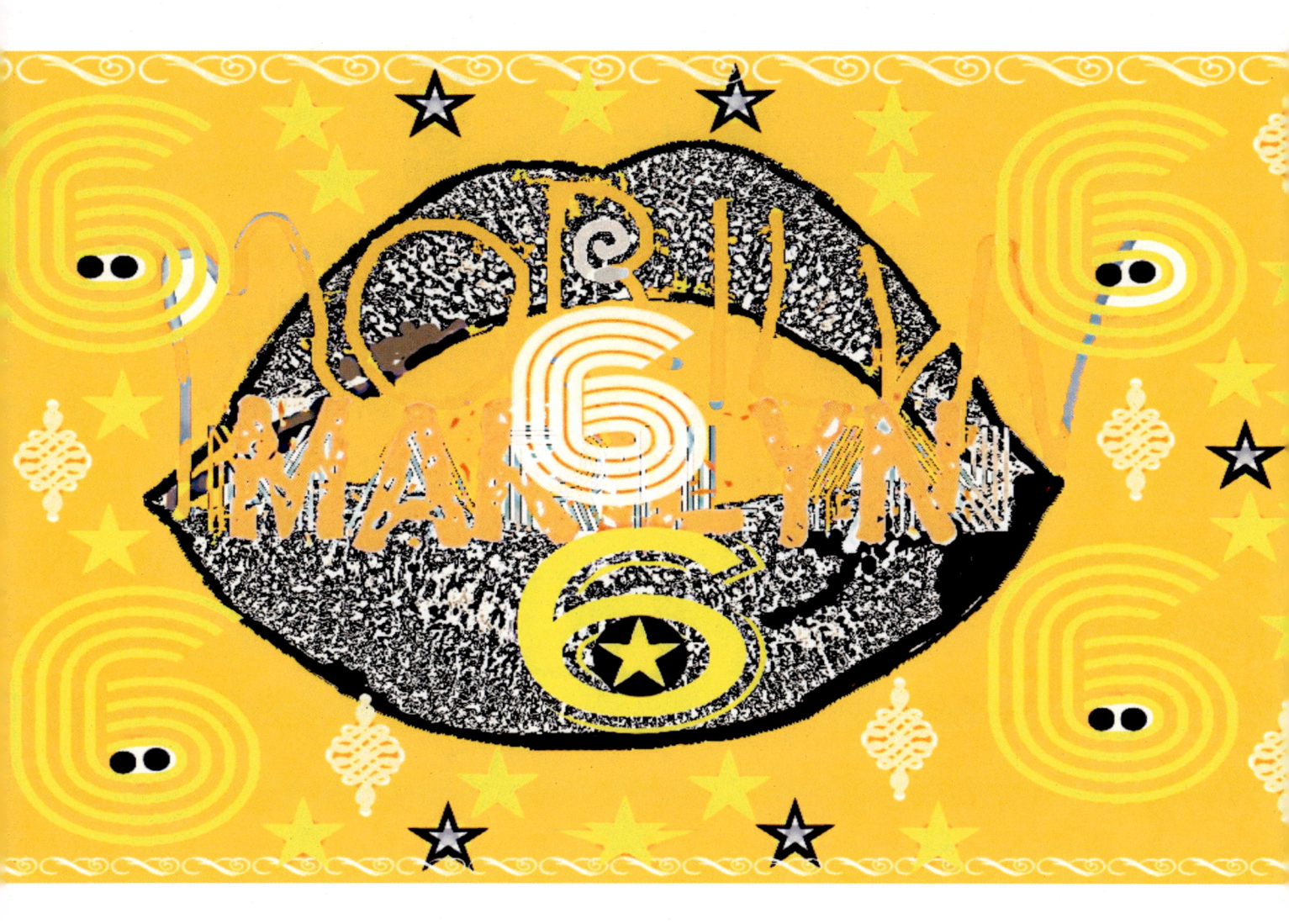

Saturn. Domestic, responsible, conventional, provider, protector Healer, idealistic, selfless honest, charitable, faithful, nurturer, truth, order economy, emotional depth, curiosity humanitarian, unselfishness, Disconnected unaware, hypocritical, moral superiority, weak unpractical, superiority complex, weak impractical balance, good provider Peaceful, self-sacrifice, empathy, sympathy unconditional love, circulation, agriculture. Balance, Grace simplicity, ability to compromise, tolerant, reliable, seeker, unselfish, cheerful. Loving Energetic, submissive shallowness, restlessness, selfishness, weak-willed, unsupportive. Very easily stressed. Compassionate, responsible, reliable, true with family, friends. Domestic self-Righteous. A slave to others, neglect own needs, thrive, supporting others. Magnetic

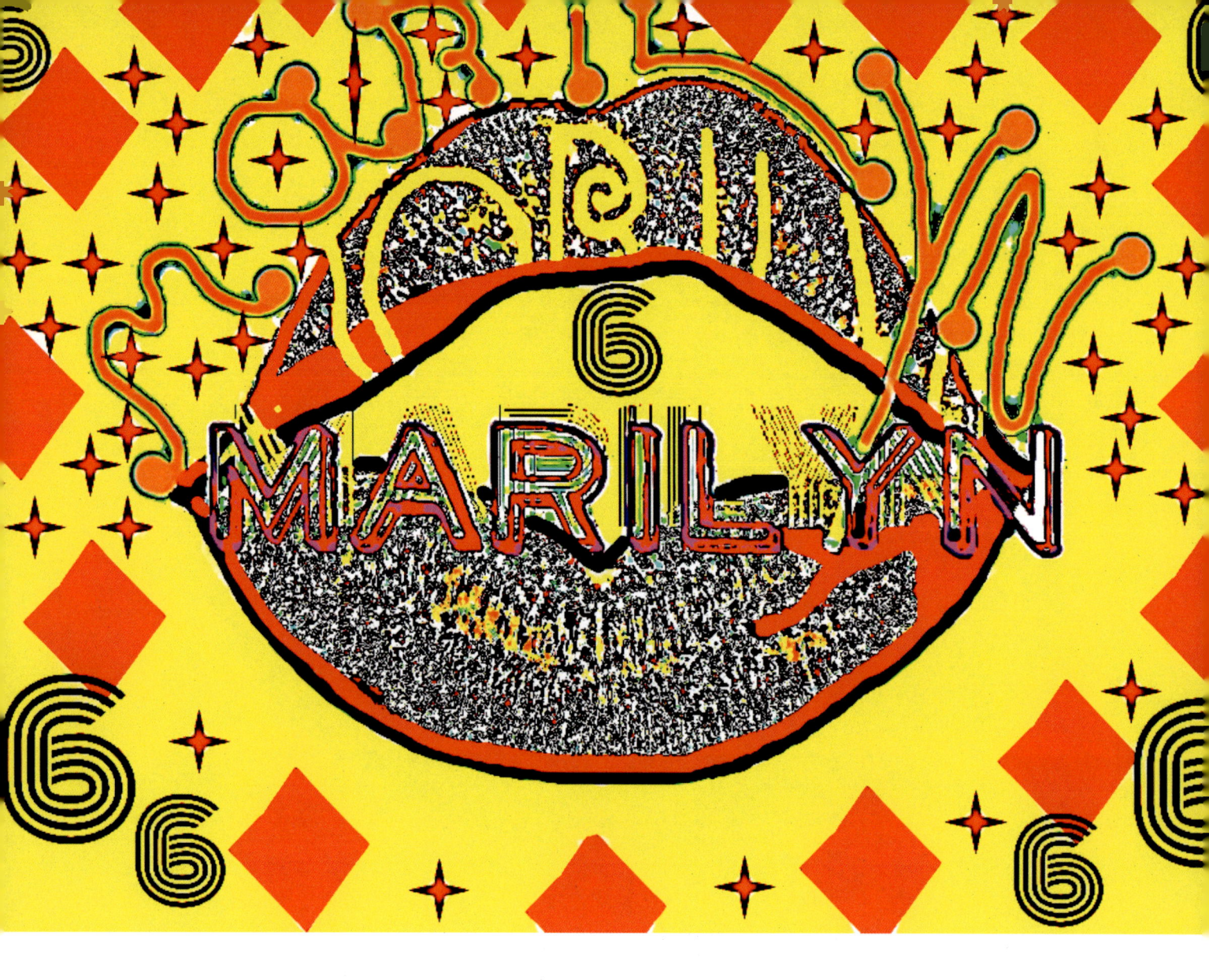

Until you came, the world was full with light

The fire burns inside of you burned anything in its path

Your devilish power, destroyed anything which doesn't bend to yours will

One day, Mr. beast. You will start to run in cycles

After your own shadows. When someone will stick a bullet inside of your head

Since you are far away from symbolized the number six

Seven

My sex oral video

Mr. president. It was not a healthy environment to bring a child to. My husband was worried our children will be kidnapped, and they will not be able to protect me and them. I could sense their inner weakness and worried, I will throw up on them in the end, for a stronger man which can protect me and my future children. There were plenty of a strong man around me waiting to have my attention. My husband had deserted me before I will abandon them for a stronger figure.

Haven't you heard out about the multimillionaire, owning my original oral sex picture video? He Paid millions of dollar bills to maintain my "honor, " I desire to ask Mr. Millionaire, in front of the Godly eyes, why did you take my video home, instead of destroying it at the present of the press? The fact, you have got so much money, to buy my oral sex video, doesn't leave any question mark what so ever, regard, what you are doing with it while acting a hot bathtub. So much honor, I find. You know, personally, I don't care what you are doing with this video. Obviously everyone knows what you are doing. Masturbating with a lot of soap.

It was much more honorable to tell the true statement. Only the truth can honor me, not more bullshit and stories. All of you the rich guys own. Why can't you say to the media: "I am most of the time suffering from impotence, I believe having sex with the late Marilyn Monroe, will be much more erotic and arisen to me, than with any living female". Can you just do it? Tell the truth to the press? Let see how brave you are, behind all your millions. It's not much to ask. Be truthful.

If anyone is buying your story about as if, saving my self-esteem, they are so naïve. You should have feed millions of children, with your money instead of buying my oral video. There are dozens of orphan children around the world to feed. Did you ever consider, millions of babies could be fed with this money, the only respect you gave by broaching this video is, to yourself, certainly not to me. The honor I deserve and want, has nothing to do with being a known figure or a sex symbol. Especially, not having a sex oral video in your hands, you watch in your house. Let's face the truth now shall we, the truth is. No one ever honor me, in the way I needed. I am bound under this rubric of the "sex symbol". Because of it, humanity had found me along my life, as a guilty of a crime. Regard my over sexuality. I being found guiltier in fact, even more than my murderer. The facts show, my sexuality is popular after my death. Because I'd rather be dead for the sake of the business makers. And you are Mr. multimillionaire is just one of them.

Image 139 page 307. Seven. Model. Painter: Dr. Marilyn Monroe. Photographer: Ofer Frohlich

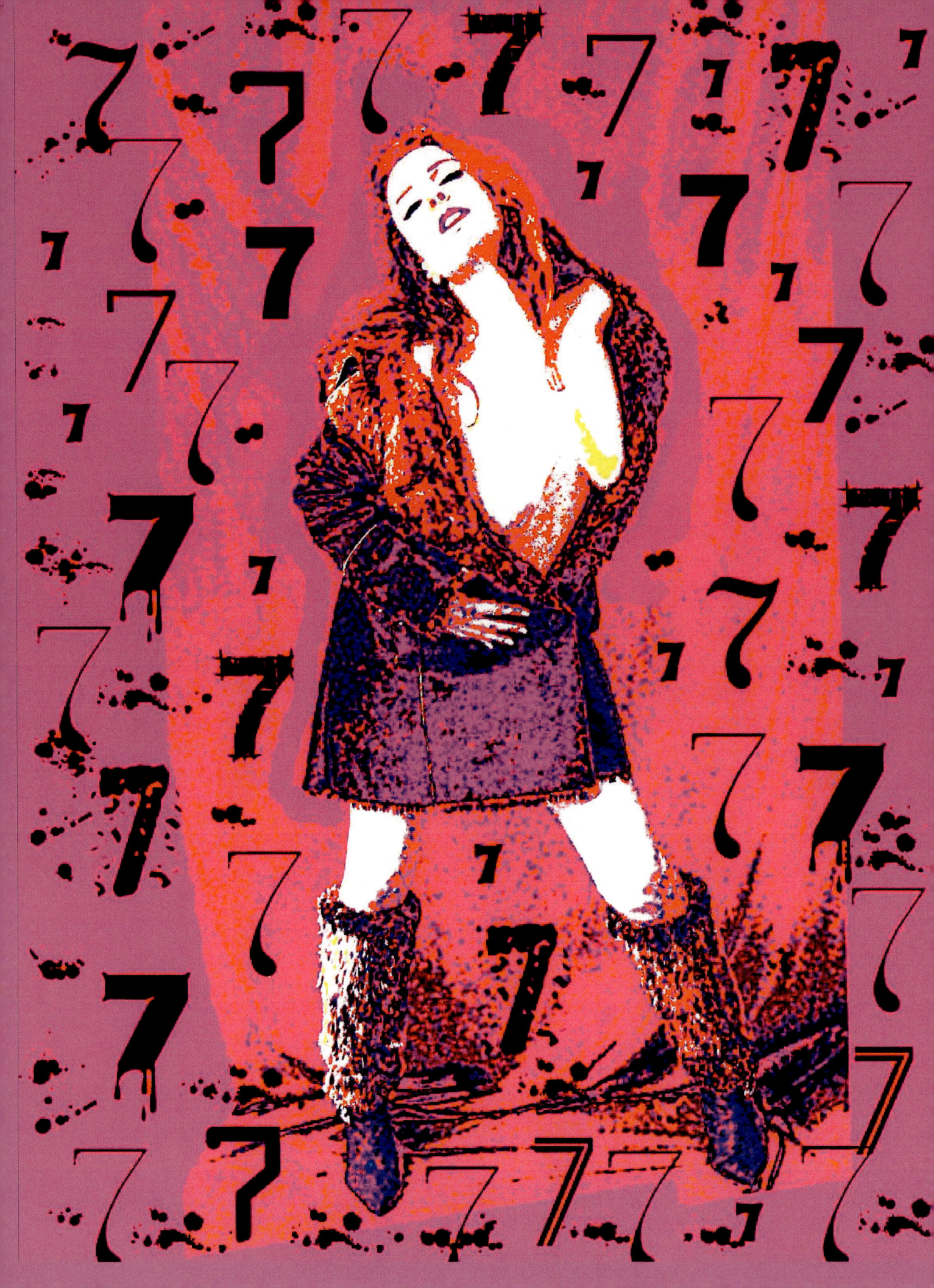

Number Seven -7 meanings

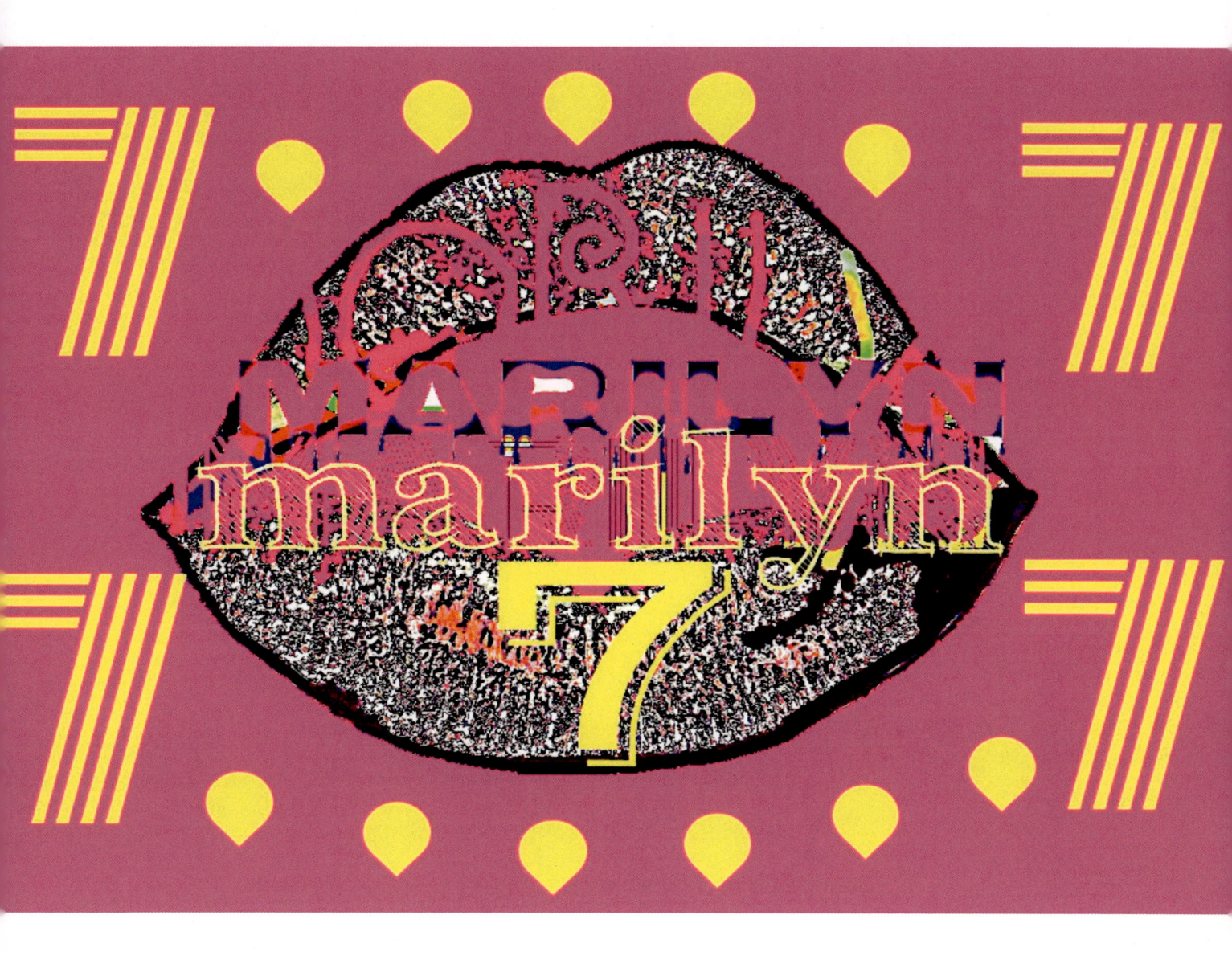

The number seven meanings: Uranus, Completeness, divine perfection, the seeker, the searcher of Truth, hidden truths. Introverted, shy, intellectual, offbeat perspective. Metaphysical, spiritual Hates gossip, Money means nothing, humor, natural love of art. Sense of justice. Tall, analyst's Strategic planners. Academics, science. Researchers' methodical analysis, have faith. Cynical ocean. Intuitive, aloof, loner, pessimistic, secretive and insecure; quiet, peaceful, solitude. Higher awareness, a wider point of view. Change mini-adventures, The seven colors of the rainbow. The Sabbath, the day God gives us – rest. The end of the creation. God

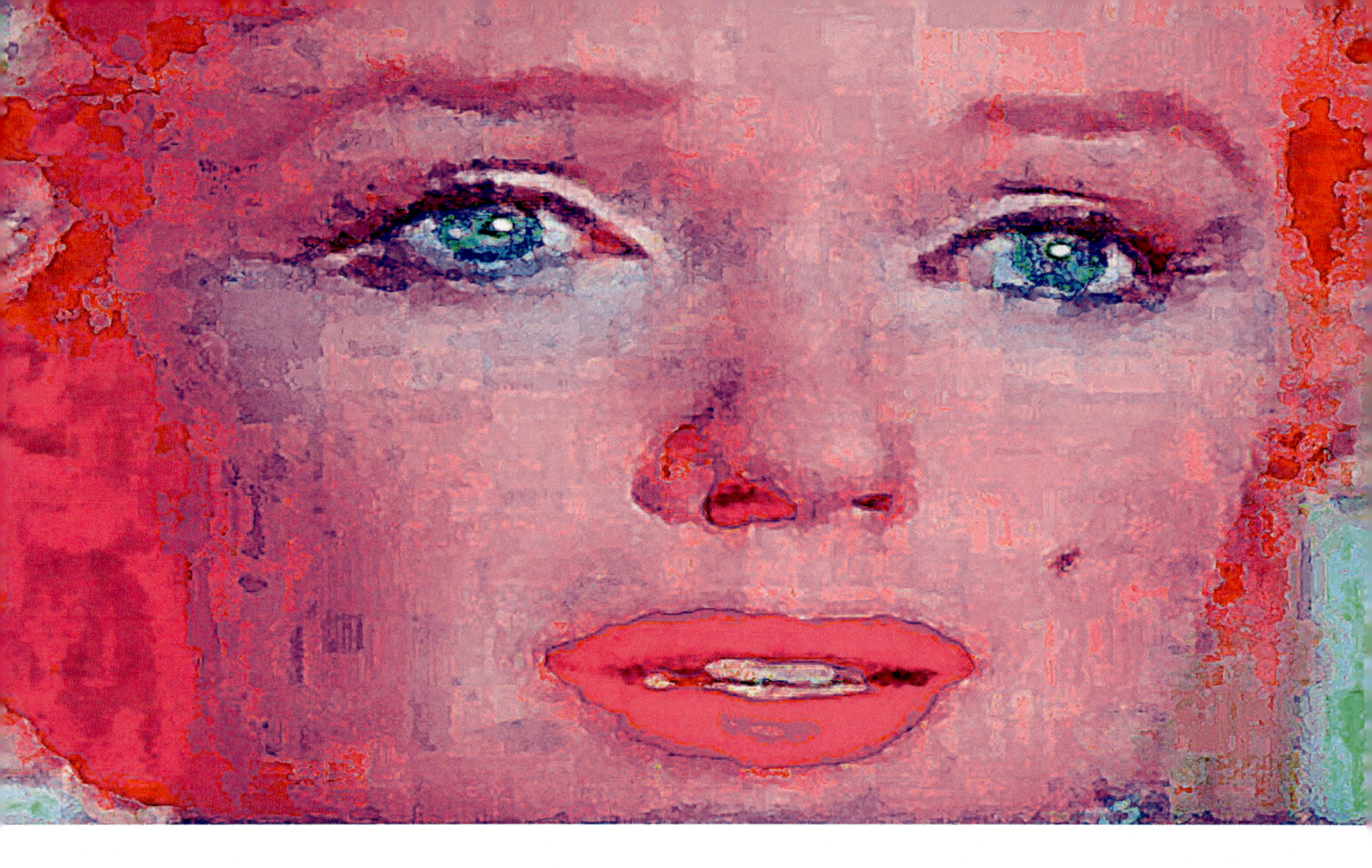

When I met you, you were strong as my heart beats.

Today I understand how weak you are

I felt secure with you from my own nightmares

But now I know you were my biggest one Inside your bed

I could dream about a better life.

Only today I recognize this future never meant to do

Beside you, I used to imagine I will never wake up at nighttime

Worried, what will happen to me when the sun will rise

It truth, now I don't have to worry.

Since I am dead. Rest in peace as you said

There is nothing to worry about, as long as I left you with all my sex video. You can Imagine… Imagine… imagines…. Imagines….. …… And explode

Eight

Sex Weekend with 100 men

Mr. President. The mafia boys planned to have a full weekend with me. 100 important men, were required to take part in the privet party, they demanded to purchase an entrance ticket, cost a thousand of dollars. The men, which paid the most, get the higher number 100. The numbers were an important part in keeping the order. The memory around a hundred men with numbers, had come with me into the presents. Around the age 3 – 4. I started to remember things from my past. Right after I revealed inside of my father's closet, my Marilyn Monroe red velvet nude image. Then, it's like opening a gate, a flow of memory and visions, in the channel of time. I start seeing myself making sex with a large group of human beings, their big organs penis was entirely all over me. White men, dark men, red men yellow men, with all sizes of tools, standing about me, waiting for their time. This visualizes I got to the age 15 years old, were coming to hunt me, every night and day. I asked my mother, Sarah, which of course I didn't reveal to her anything, I didn't want to shock her, but I ask for her to get a psychological assistance. Can you tell me, where these images are coming from into a little girl's head at the age 3-15 years old? Thanks god, I knew to express myself toward art, or else, I could explode. A heavy burden on a little girl's. According to the true facts I was after, around my investigation of my murder scene as: Norma Jean. Marilyn Monroe, I had found out, it's possible for a little child, to remember her past life, in it, she was sexual abused, even if she were at that time, under an Anastasia manipulation. Under the mixture of a "rape drugs" the men tool manipulations. https://en.wikipedia.org/wiki/Date_rape_drug. Which allow men to ride on her for hours, while she is not under a full awakened state, sleeping or losing awareness. What's amazing is: the soul, is witness to all the events fully, if a woman will be hypnotized, the soul will bring out all the clear facts, and memory into the sour face. She will know precisely, what took place with her, who was in the room, what they did, as if she was fully awake. This same ability is known in people, which are in the coma state of mind and soul. https://en.wikipedia.org/wiki/Coma. Or as well people under a near death experience https://en.wikipedia.org/wiki/Near-death_experience. Everybody thinks this person is under a deep sleep, don't hear nothing, see nothing, not aware of nothing, but they do, fully. There are a plenty of medical research, and information, around this topic. At the age 10, at this present, I start to paint what I saw, in my daydreaming. I didn't see it on TV, at that time sex, was not at all popular in the press, as it is today 46 years later. My parents have purchased, the first white and black with no channels TV machine, while I was around 7-8 years old. My family was a kind of a Jewish religious bound family, sexuality, was not at all a topic in our life. No one talk about it, in any kind of way. It was mysterious.

Image 140 page 311. Eight. Model. Painter: Dr. Marilyn Monroe. Photographer: Ofer Frohlich

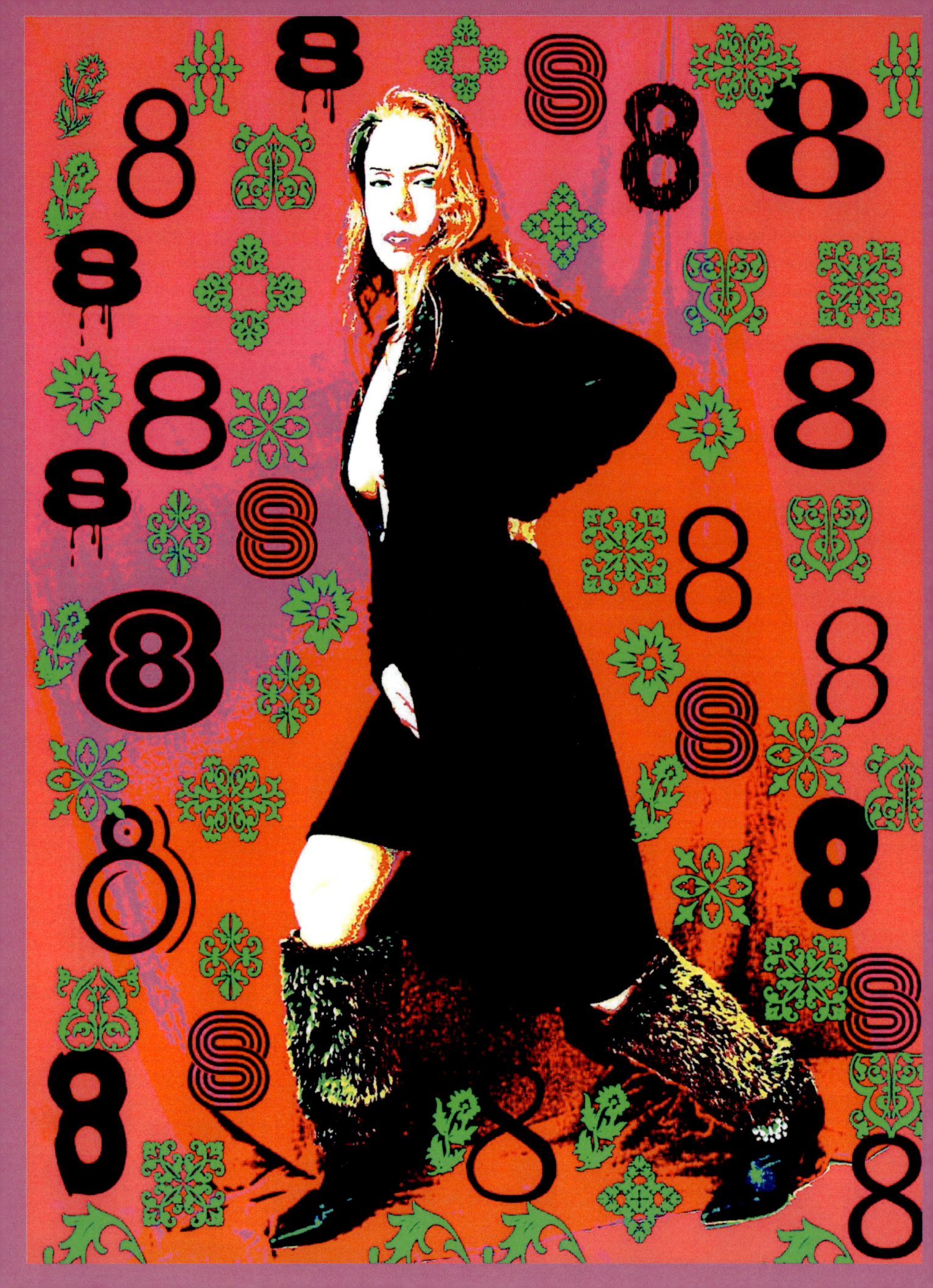

As a little child, you bear pure into your new life, regard the understanding of your sexuality. Therefore, I did not know exactly how to interpret, what these visuals of sex means. I was thinking these men are dancing with me. When you are rebirth into a new life as a kid, your memory and understanding, regarding what sex is, is very limited back to the understanding of a youngster. You are coming back with a fresh, natural, pure knowledge about sexuality. But at the back of my mind. My Marilyn Monroe soul, I got. I knew exactly what this vision means, I knew everything about sex from the first day I was born again. This information from the past, start attracted men to me, the same as it did when I was 36 years old in my last year of life as Marilyn Monroe. Simply, they felt I was alive, inside of this little girl's new body, their soul was fully aware, of my refresh, and new existence at the present, as a sex symbol of all times. Naturally, they wanted to touch me.

This sexuality visions, day dreaming. Made me start masturbate from the years 3 - 4 and I couldn't stop. These images had kept running inside of my inner vision, I could watch these men, as well feel them, as if, we are making love in the reality, it was that real. Because I was a little child, I didn't cognize how to enterprise my visions fully, since, the Lord, protect us from all the knowledge we had inside of us, from our past lives. Therefore, I got an innocent look on this vision, knowing and not knowing at the same time, what's taking place with me and with this man. Until the age 12 years old. I saw in the dictionary at school, the word "masturbation". I was extremely embarrassed. I instantly knew, I was necessitated in some sort of a criminal offense.

In real life, men could not prevent themselves with touching me, asking me to keep it in secret. The same secret feeling enveloped me from my past, rolled over into the present. I was asked to be cooperative. I did, I was an obedient naïve girl, exactly as I did, in my past. At the age 5 I was mature regard sexual secrets, This De Ja Vu state of mind, capture my attention. The interest around me and the secretive attitude, made me feel significant important. But I was just a little girl, this adventure which came with me from the past, were heavy on my little shoulder made me collapse. Not once. But millions of times in a raw. Finally, the knowledge which was transferred to me from my past. Regard being a sex symbol, a tool to have sex with, no more. Side by side to the fact, I was an extremely phenomenal talented, extremely much more than just a body to share.

The understanding I am still being locked inside of this fake prison of the sex symbol, haunted by these prejudice idea men enveloped me with, since they could capable of seen just my overall enveloped. I felt my reborn was a spell. I just wished, I would have never been reborn again into this world. That doesn't deserve to have me inside, m as a high spiritual value.

Number Eight - 8 meanings

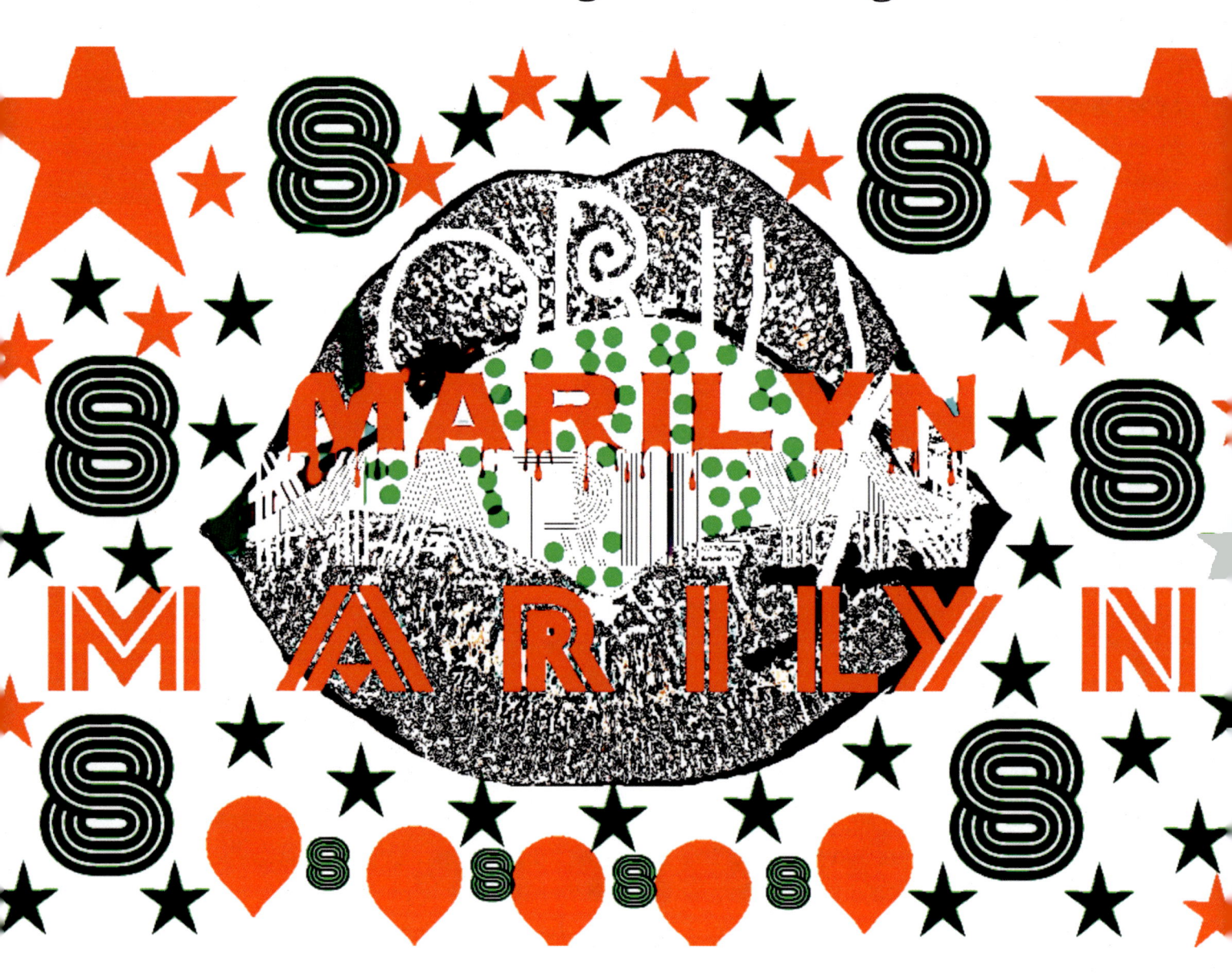

Neptune, strong intuition, insight, mild, honest, hides their real emotions, philanthropic generous, leadership qualities, abundant ambitions. Courage, sincerity Decent, fascinating reliable. Self-centered, arrogant. Encourage people, potential. Don't worry Enthusiastic. Sacrifice. Spiders have eight legs. The octopus has eight arms. Mathematical symbol for infinity. The birth of the Virgin Mary September 8. Jesus showed himself alive 8 times after his resurrection from the dead. A new beginning, a new order, a new creation, resurrected from the dead into eternal life. Authority, material wealth, very ambition, and very caution.

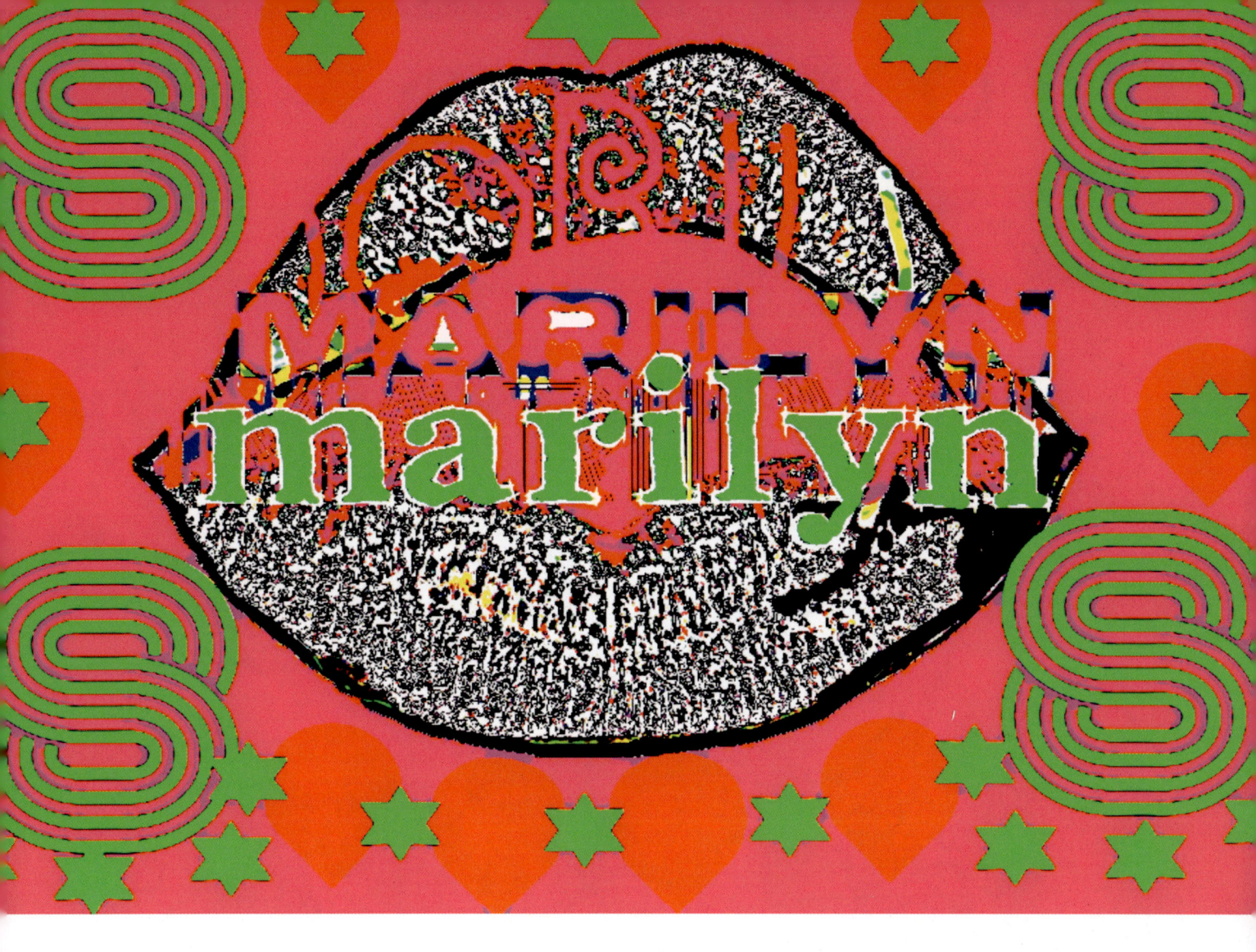

I am Lolita. Innocence child inside of a barbarian world.

I had no place to escape to. To retain the quiet, I used to feel at heart

No way to run, nowhere to hide. If I wanted to go, it was only, back into your open arms

As you used to dance with me all night inside of the dark. Dancing to the rhythm of music.

At the first time we made that dance, when my blood passed into the sheet, you told me that all right, Since You got a big bodyguard between your legs.

It looks like a hot dog; you teach me how to corrode. You said this body guard need to keep both of us together forever. This is why, he is getting in and out very fast, he need to check that everything is all right. I believed you, what else could I do?

No way to hide. Only inside of my heart, Jesus. Doesn't like what you had done.

Image 141 page 315. Nine. Model. Painter: Dr. Marilyn Monroe. Photographer: Ofer Frohlich

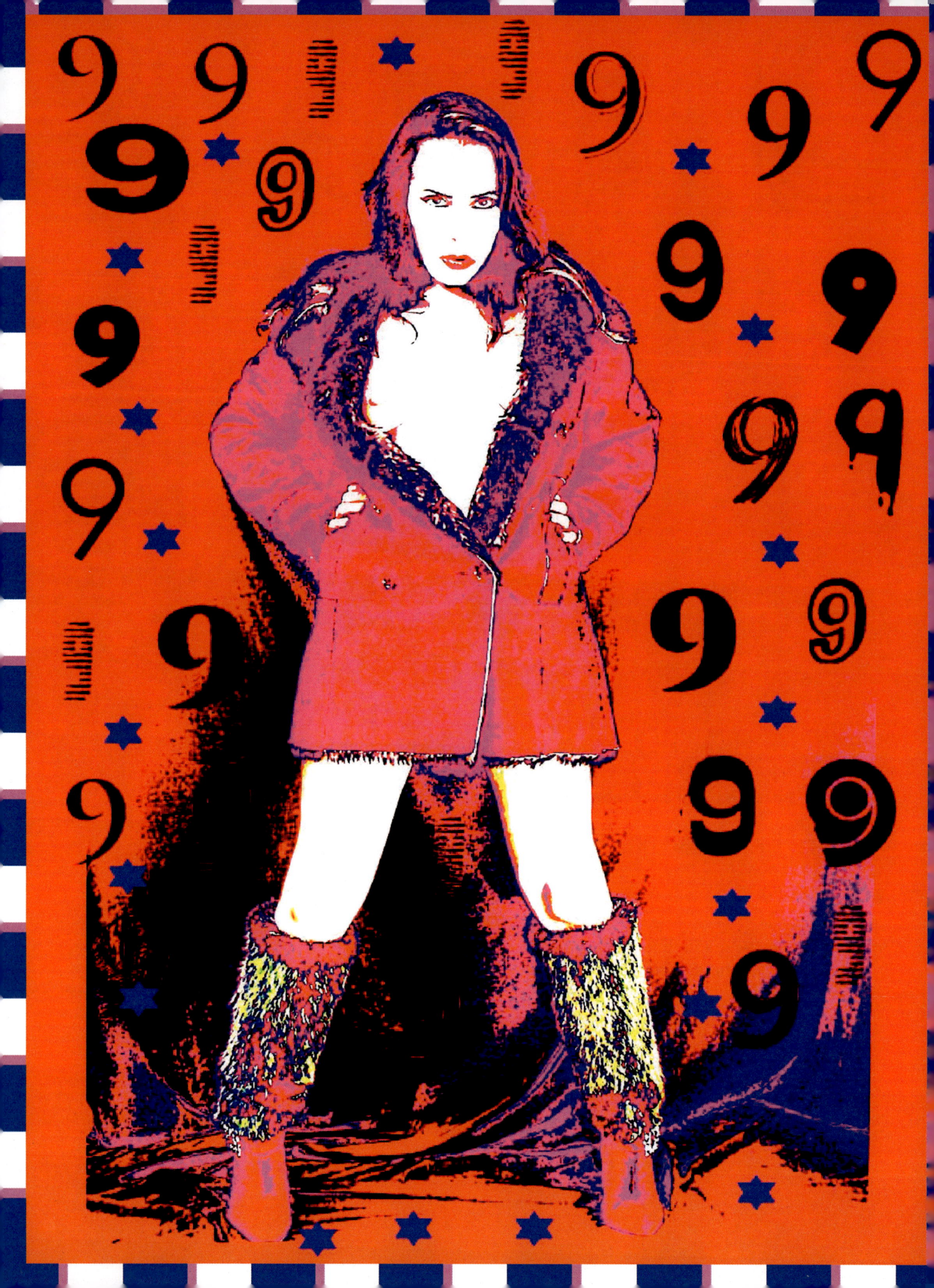

Nine

The hunted soul

Mr. President. From a young age, I knew to draw horses, as if I lived with them all my life. Only. Along this present life, I never got the chance to be near a real horse. Amazingly, I knew how to portray them exactly as they were. Since I got a De JA Vu from the motion picture "The misfit". The last movie I was part in of Arthur Miller my husband. I always felt horse are more human than human. I draw them endlessly; from the day I could express myself in this lifetime. There were days around the age 6 - 12 years old. I am painting one after the other endless forms of horses. Standing. Running. Jumping. Falling. The falling horse trying to stick up. Is one of my favorite paintings. I always felt this horse is telling my life story, reminded me of my past. https://en.wikipedia.org/wiki/The_Misfits_(film)

Around the age 7, I used to star long minutes, at a certain point at a corner of the wall. While I was daydreaming visions was coming up. It was like looking at a film running in front of my eyes. I felt mesmerized by these sights. I looked at them, recognize myself inside. I used to question myself: if I am here looking at this visual sensation and see myself there, how can it be I am in both places at the same time? Sitting and looking at myself there. At the age 14 I start posing in full nude in front of different photographers. It was not an everyday scene in 1985. But for me, it was a Continue from the same spot I left behind in my past life. It was not odd. It was doing something usual, I used to do and experienced with. My nude photos relived inside of me, my past memories. Tamla Yalin, an art school, was the place I start reliving my past life nude art, nude portrait myself. Finally, I get in touch, with the Tom Kelley studio again, in order to relive my red velvet nude art with him. I start to create endless pose on the scarlet velvet with different photographers.

One more thing kept hunted me from the past. It was a natural hilarious state of mind, "as if" I was on drugs, but I wasn't. We got rules in my parents' house to be strict about drugs. No. was the only answer I gave, when drugs offered to me at the present. I instantly was against it. Later one, inside of the homeopathic school. I learned drugs have a mental and physical state they are creating in the individual. In the concluding weeks of my life as Marilyn, I was enveloped with so many drugs. Their side effect follows me into the present. Being funny, easy going. Laughing, mocking, making nonsense, facial expressions, dancing, being sexual energetic. No boundaries. Where the side effect of the drugs, I was given in the past. I needed to clean myself from, which I did toward the homeopathy. These drugs caused me lose my individuality. Dr. Greenson. Was not intimate with other methods. I become a reflection of another person's identity and will. My sub conscience memory of my murder, keeps reminding me, drugs are equal to death.

Number Nine - 9 meaning

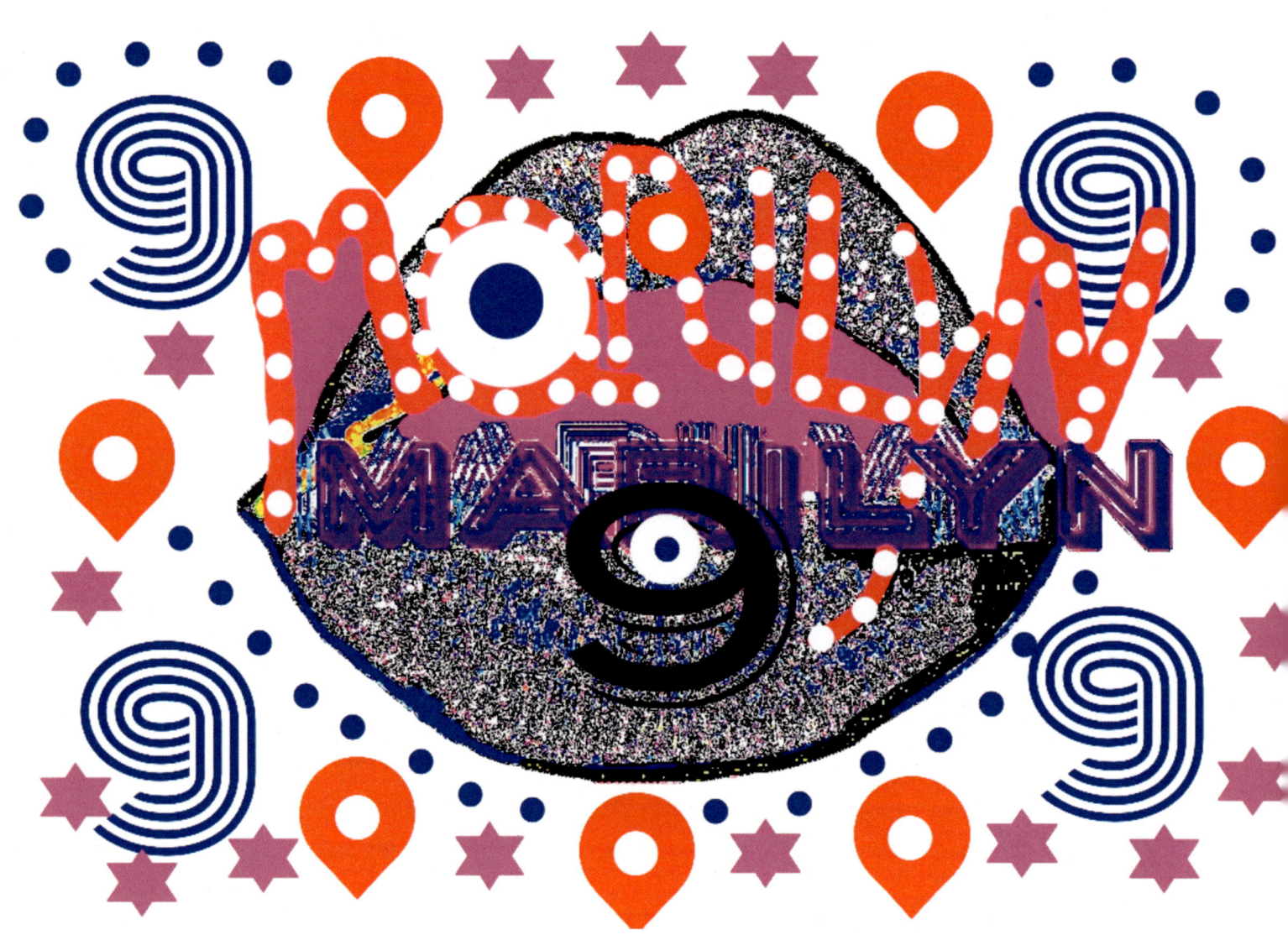

Faithfulness, Gentleness, Goodness, Joy, Kindness, long suffering Love. Peace and Self-control. Finality. Christ died in the 9th hour of the day, or 3 p.m., to make the way of salvation open to everyone. Brilliant, funny, smart and generous. Humanitarians Compassion Generosity. A full spiritual light consciousness. A light working and Light workers philanthropy, charity, self. Sacrifice, destiny, a higher perspective, romance, inner-strength responsibility intuition, creative. Loyalty, brilliance, problem-solving, freedom, popularity tolerance, altruism benevolence, Conformity, genius, an expansive viewpoint, an eccentricity communication perfection. the last month of the pregnancy, the start a beginning.

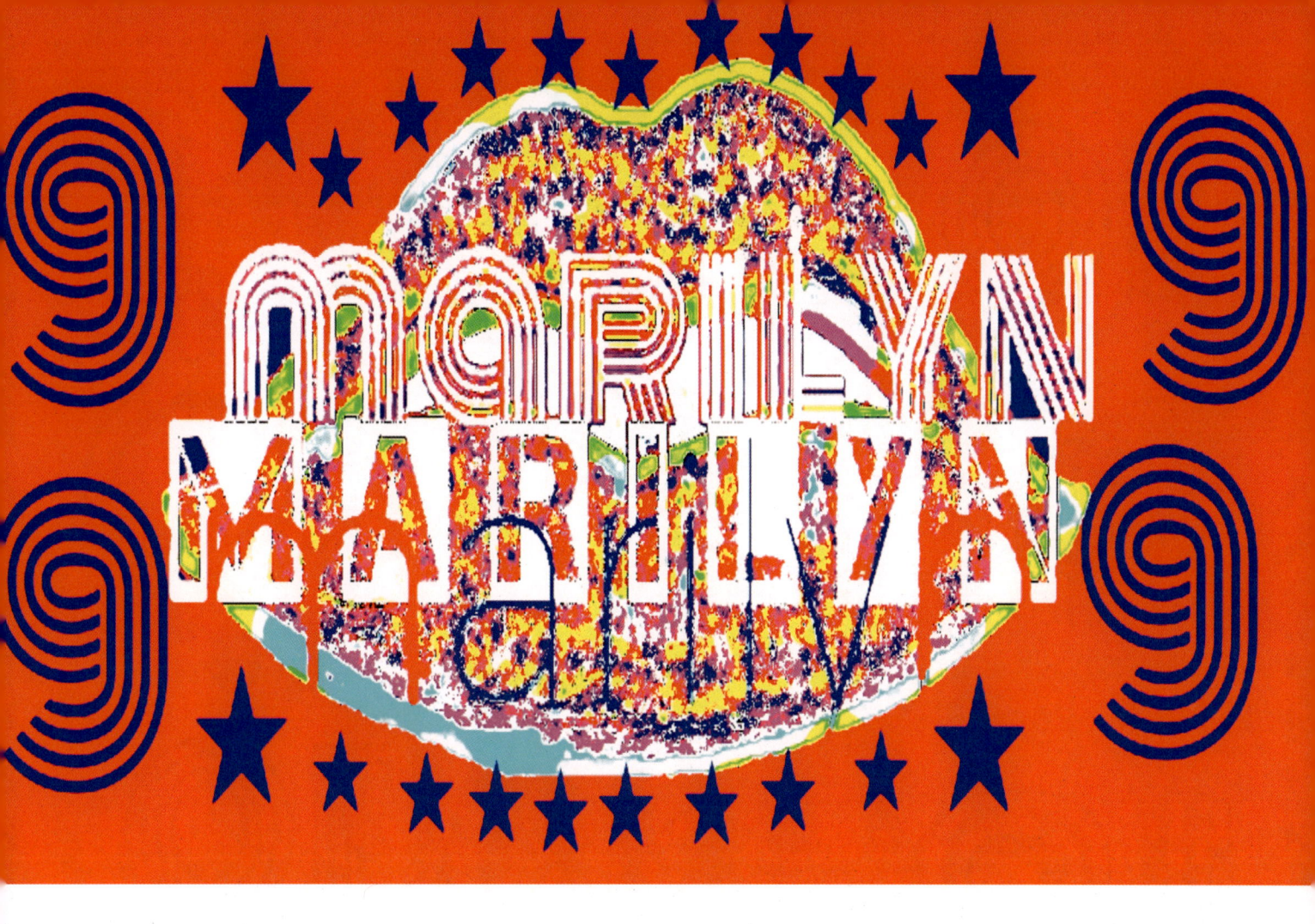

The drugs stop me of feeling my true core. I become enveloped with clouds

My brain kept fighting, but it cells stops cooperating with me

Like a conspiracy against myself from the inside of my brain cells

I had forgotten for a while, all the injuries and wounds I carry on my back

The essence of my desire for life, my ability to put my head up, against any drug

Made me start to live again. Knowing who I am and what I am worth

While my creator was looking at me from above

Every day I promised the lord, I will make one more little step, forward toward his light

Eventually I will conquer my brain. My soul. My Life.

If you are holding the faith around the lord

He will hold your hand back. Don't forget to breath. Nine times in and out.

Image 142 page 319. Ten. Model. Painter: Dr. Marilyn Monroe. Photographer: Ofer Frohlich

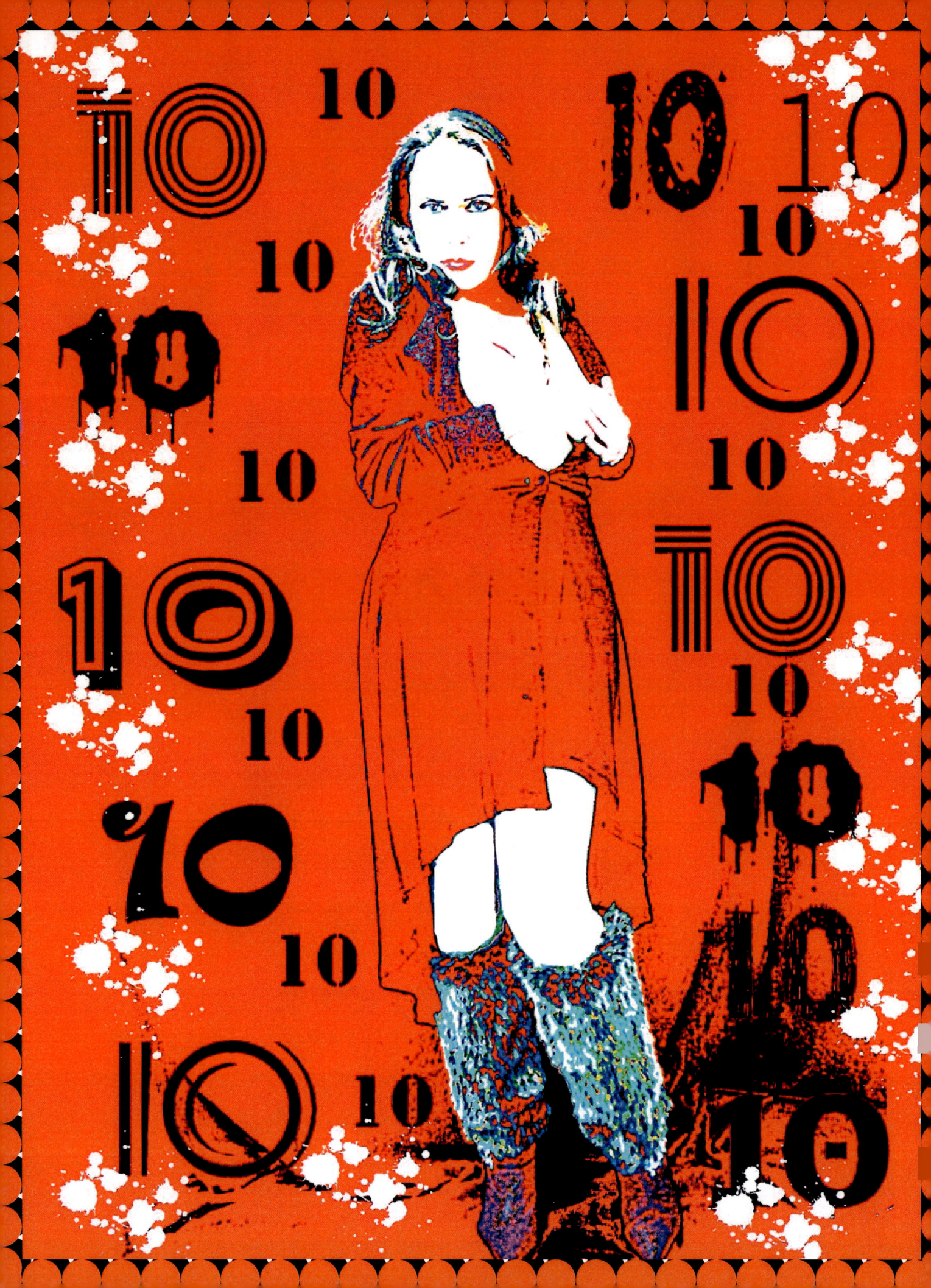

Ten

Last weekend with Marilyn

Mr. President. I really hate this chapter, this chapter makes me feel sick, terrible, a victim. I wish I could avoid writing it, but I can't, I must do it. You know, at the editing process, at the end of the editing of the book, while I was working on the last corrections, suddenly I realized this chapter is missing. No 10 was not there. This is a sign: you may not want to read this chapter, if you do, you will know my soul deeper then you do know. But it will be a painful process. As you can see, I came back with a full compensation. A full command over my mind and soul, an internal natural awareness around: losing a control on my brain, by drugs alcohol, or any medicine. Will take me into a calamitous end of life. Side by side to it, my artwork kept revealing secrets from my past. From around the age 13 years old, my paintings become distressing, kept enveloped remain me, my last Marilyn day.

I painted them and then, I want to tear them apart. My nude tormented body and soul, were the chief part inside of my art, contain a secret body languish, predictably, revealing secrets from my past. It was like a mirror, I looked inside every day, and watch the script of my past life running in front of me, like the script of all your life, which is flowing in front of your eyes when you are going. When I was naked, in front of the camera, my body movement was divulged intimacy secrets from within my hidden soul, it was a cry for help, but no one could hear it...

My past dying process as Marilyn, unfolds toward my body language movements. You can see it in my videos. These videos I made around the last 10 years, enveloped the torment I had been in. It is written all over my body and face, you can see there a woman struggling with a deadly kind of process. It's like a woman caught inside of a Giant Octopus arm trying to escape. Trying to sort out, but she can't, my voice is not being heard on this video. Just the movement of my body and the expression of my face, are distressing.

It reminds me a bit of Amy Winehouse on one of her stage performances while she was on drugs. You can see death is there in her eyes, in her face and body expressions. And again, I was not on drugs. In this present life I had never taken any drug. It's the state of mind, my body and face revealing toward art, each time I was in front of the camera of the present, my expressions revealed what took place with me in my past. What hidden secrets my soul is crying, tormented by. Without any out late, just toward my artistic creation, I could speak and give an out late to it. Let's come back to the conductors of my party shell we. This people, the manager behind this scene of my party were, a sophisticate animal with a sophisticated animal's brain. One of the basic drugs they fed me with was: a laughter drug. This drug kept me cheerful, I become obsessed with making of a stupid mimic, an uncontrollable spasm, and tics shown up in my typeface. I was laughing, from any stupid move or expression made by myself or others. I totally lost it, I was not myself anymore, couldn't pick out myself. I become the entertainment of the show. Since nobody desires to lose my clownish charm. Tickets were sold for this "final cut show with Marilyn". This animal, human, was eager to be with their privet queen, saint, slut, servant, love one, sweetheart, have the best sex they could ever dream of. I was the Prey booty of a manhood victory. Half dragged half drunk, no way, I could escape. Far out from being under a full conciseness, or even acknowledge who I am. The primary grounds, of course, for satisfying me with this specific drug of laughter were: Their need to prevent from me, to interfere their party by: begging's, crying, shouting, it didn't conform with their festival.

One more benefit they received with the help of this drug side effect was: the fact it made me become sexual arousal thousand times more, than I used to be. Whether I wanted it or not, my sexual drive, become extremely high, I become an extremely nymphomaniac, it was completely not in my hand to terminate it, or hold it. The drug effect took a perfect command over my existence. I was occupying the air of the room with a full energy of a sexual arousal hormone, it was a blessing for all the ticket buyers, there were plenty of men to feed, to roll with me on the red velvet, like a cigarette chewing inside of their lip and hands. I was rolled over and over again and again, from one into another, being sexual assault endlessly. "Smile Marilyn smile for me", "smile for me Marilyn, smile, yes, smile for me, I am coming" Marilyn smile I am coming" oh yes yes yes smile, smile, smile Marilyn, Marilyn... They repeated it in my ears, penetrating me, like an echo. Everyone needs my smile. Even when I am being tormented.

My body, was too expensive to fill with it my grave, to allow the little worms to be fed with. I consider the original body of mine, is not buried inside of my tomb. I hope one day, the government of the USA, will manage to order of a checkup of a DNA to the body buried inside of my tomb, to help determine, if the body which is buried inside of it is genuinely mine, or of a look-alike me. It is obvious today, my murders, had knew my body received an extremely rare value. Been estimated, as one of the largest and most precious diamond, that had ever created on that plant. You believe, Mr. president. They could let me disappear just like that, being eaten by a white virgin worm? While each bite and peace of my nude body flesh and skin, is equal to "money" money" money" money gold diamonds" lots of diamonds". No way, a conspiracy had been always around my body, long time before I found my death, and I knew it.

Now, let go back, to the man was in charge of preparing my body. He has one blue eye. I think I already told you, he was missing his left eye. Due to the Vietnam War. A sculpture I made at the age 22 at my present life, is presenting his face with one eye only. He revealed to me, how he will make a Stuff – mummy out of me. Explained me in details, how will he transfer me into an amazing as if alive Marilyn - mummy. In parliamentary law, to hold my body clean, young forever as he need to, as a Marilyn Mummy piece of artwork. Him as the greatest expert in the world in this field, know how to take guardianship of my body, transfer it into a mummy, in a clean fashionable manner. Essentially, I think, my cleaning obsession today, is very much connected to him. Since he had taught me all about, how he cleans a body from the inside of it. On another body of a young beautiful female body, which was lying there, already dead. Along with cleaning my body from my outside, he could not keep his mouth shut. He accepted the need to prepare me, like a doctor before a great operation. He discloses all the facts around my coming death. But before I will alter into a mummy, I had to attend to all their sexual requirements. Poor man, he needs to keep me clean after any sex with those humans. Since I didn't have a control on my digestion. I was helpless, under a schizophrenic, a multi personality kind of state. Couldn't know who I am any longer. One portion of my brain was under a dreadful, doomed, shock state around my coming death. The other, was forced to laugh by the misuse of these drugs. I could not recognize myself anymore. It was not Marilyn me as I recognize myself, or you are familiar with. I was as if I am being controlled by some kind of entity, toward the worth spell you can imagine. Which was playing with my body and soul.

Number Ten - 10 meanings

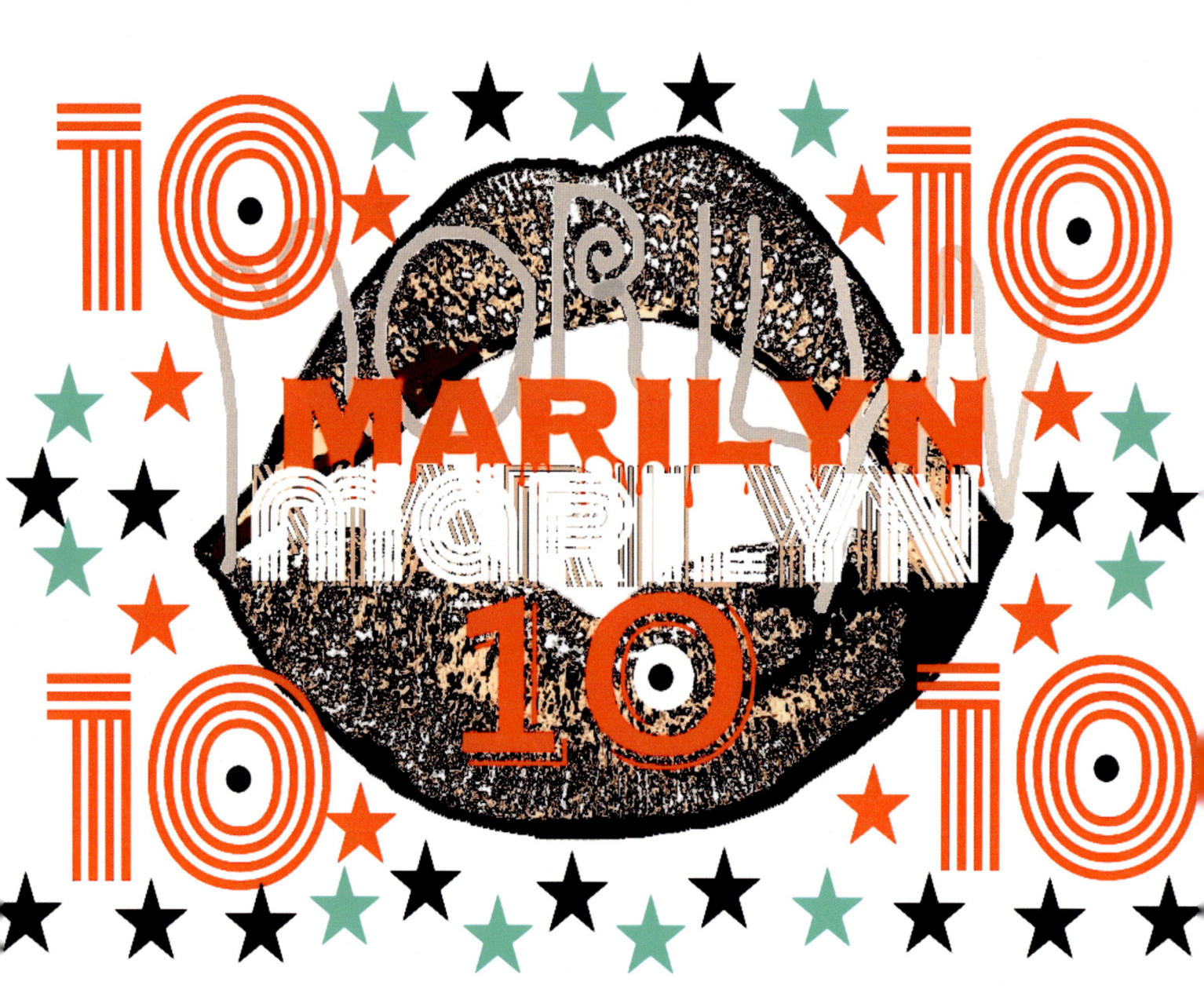

The Ten Commandments. Completion or perfection. Ten fingers. Ten toes 10 generations lived up to the flood of Noah's. 10 "I AM's" spoken by Jesus in the Gospel of John Optimism, confidence, creative powers, success, originality, adaptability, individuality, leadership Success, determination. The will of heaven and the supreme law. The highest score possible in Olympic competitions. Neon - atomic number is 10. Completion of a cycle. Integrity fullness, a return to unity. Kingdom of God, inside of Heaven. Adam-Eve. Eternity. Love and harmony inside.

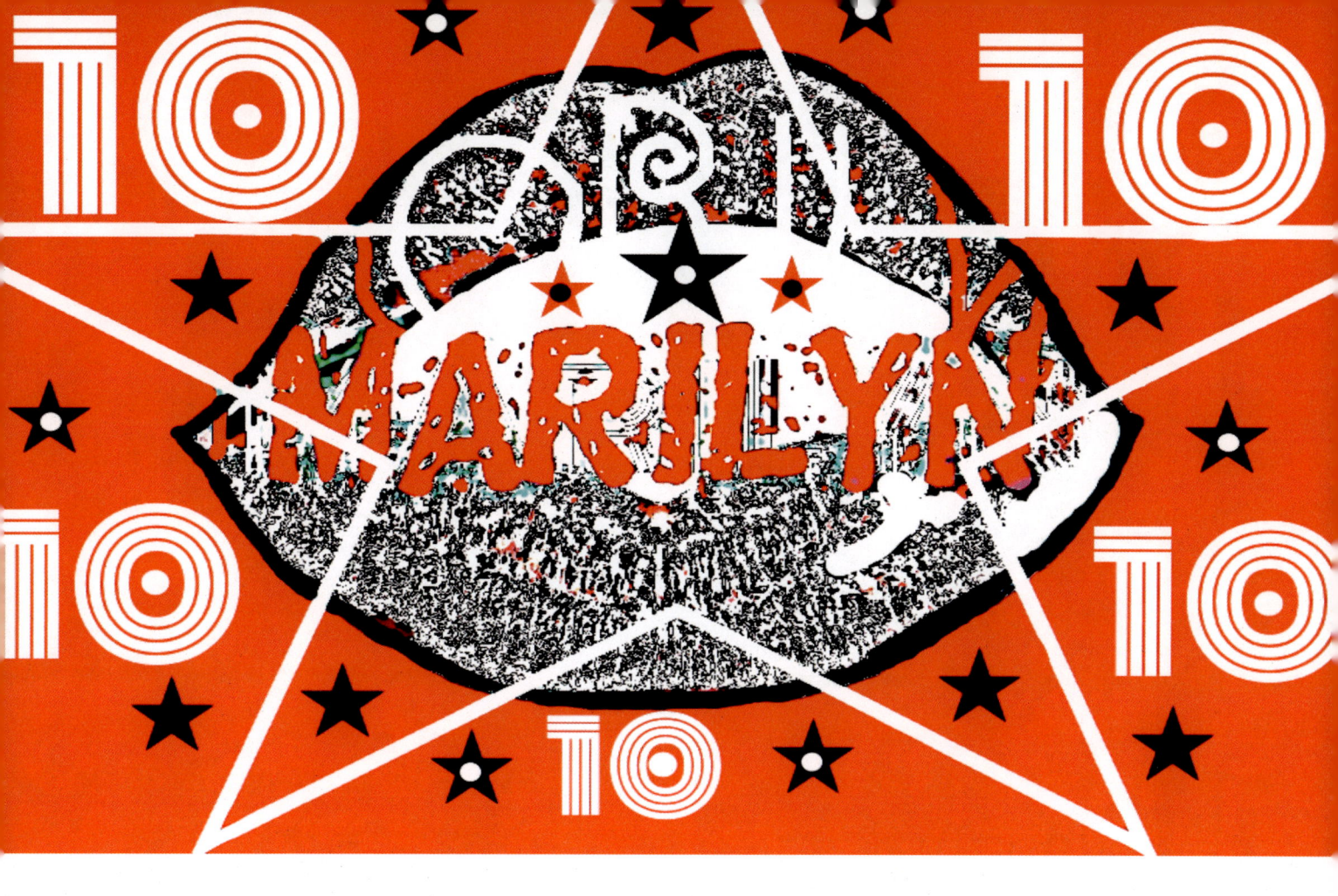

I am your privet mummy. I smile as you want.

I am your beautiful princess, hanging along your walls.

If you want to look into my blue eyes all day, they will look at your back without stop.

I am your Marilyn mummy; I will always be going to smile as you want.

Hung Side by side to the lion the tiger, and the giraffe on your walls.

They don't talk too much, and they snore at night. I am wait for you every day around the clock, to hear your voice. How are you today Marilyn? What a lucky girl you are

Up up high in the sky, my soul will grow old. Only for you, I will forever remain Virgo.

Don't forget to kiss me for a good night. I may one day come back to life.

Wake up from the dead, crawl down from the wall

lay beside you in bed. When you will wake up, it looks like, I will have to pump your heart. Don't be afraid my boy it, I was just staring at you when you snored.

Image 143 page 325. Eleven. Model. Painter: Dr. Marilyn Monroe. Photographer: Ofer Frohlich

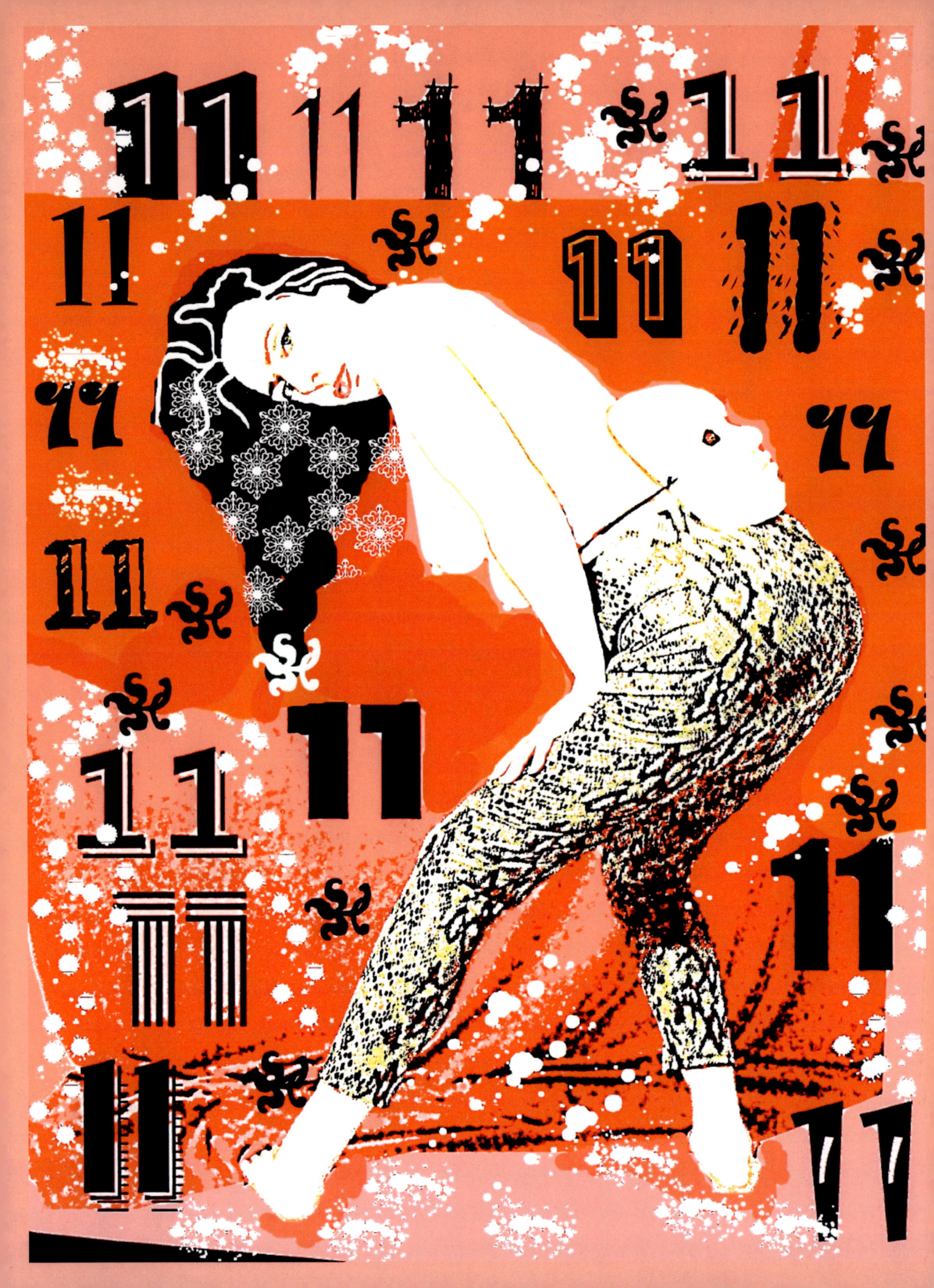

Eleven

The prince and my head statue

Mr. President. I wanted to escape, but I was paralyzed from too many drugs. The only thing my soul could do is try to escape with my soul from my body. The Duke, the one eyed man, told me: someone already paid for my head mummy, he is not less than, a real prince, a true prince. My head statue was designed to be performed as a sculpture, in his private secretive museum. This is a great honor he adds. I was "so happy" to hear, he didn't want my brain to be separated from the rest of my body. So Lucky he got a brain inside of the head. He offered few millions of dollars, in order to buy the rest of my body from all the other buyers, to save my body as one-piece artwork, taking care not to spoil my beauty. It's only because I am Marilyn Monroe, I obtained this award....

Around the age 18 years old, In one of my visits at the hospital of my mother Gladys. I revealed to her, I wanted to paint. She didn't even look at me. Then, when I bought my last house, the Brentwood. It had the right atmosphere to let me create my own art in it. To hang my paintings on my walls, was a dream come true! I adored how the impressionist had captured movement together with Light, expressing their soul toward their drawing. I desired to be able to bring life toward colors on the canvas. To make my own hand work. Which is, what I am doing eventually at this present life. At the same age of this present life, I made a sculpture, of a head, on an alabaster white stone, my love one at that age, Mathanya Abramson, brought me this stone especially from Italy. The head is a mixture, of the Duke one eye man, together with the prince and his fez on his head, together with my own self portrait. I love this sculpture very much.

Let's go back to the Duke. I was under the laughter drugs influence, one part of my brain was thinking positive, how I will be exhibited, like the famous Michael Angelo sculptures "David the Kind" what a big accolade. I always knew from a young age; I am a rare piece of a Godly Art Immortal creation. To be presented as a living forever piece of art, was a great honor. Merely, the other side of my brain, was aware I am drugged, it tried to find a way out. Is the prince being married? I asked. No. the Duke answered:

The prince is not married, but I want to assure you, it is for your own benefit, to not be marriage to the prince, you rather be his mummy, exhibit inside of his art museum, for your own benefit. You don't want to be his wife. But why? Has he been a kind of a monstrous? No. answer came from the Duke side. Why will the prince, want to have me dead instead of alive, smiling in bed every night and in the morning ready for him when he heats up. Is it because what Tony Curtis said about me: "To kiss Marilyn is like kissing Hitler"? I guess, I will never know the true answer to it.

Number Eleven – 11 meanings

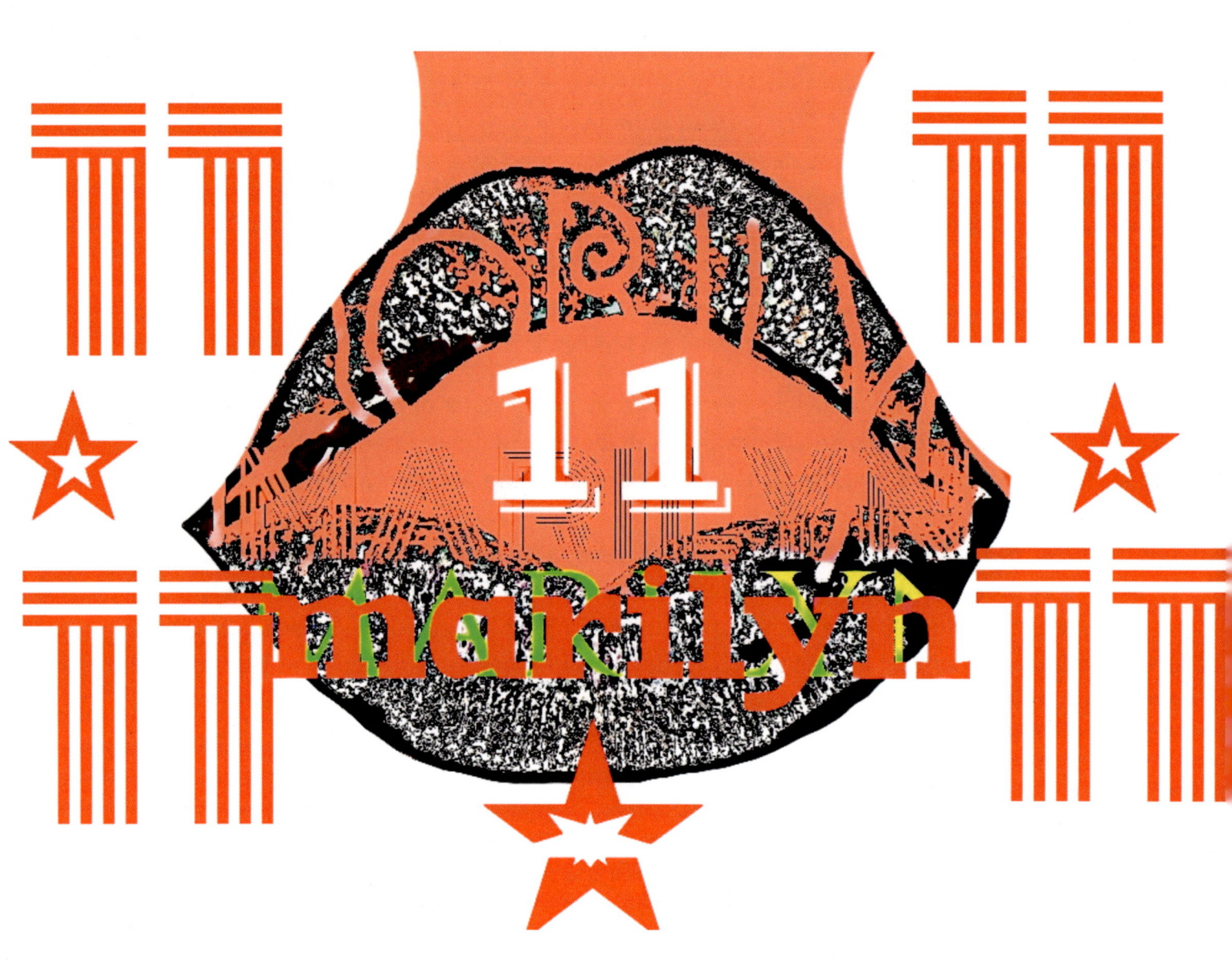

Purity presidents, politicians, managers, inspiration, enlightenment two candles, huge dreams seem unattainable kindness and friendship hypersensitivity openness Suicidal tendencies, empathy, understanding, seek freedom, love nature, animals sensual Attractive, passionate spiritual, visionary, inspiring, indecisive, impractical, nervous, overwhelmed, gift visionary individuals, psychics, mystics, healers, writers. Musicians expression, dreamer, revolution, drugs, alternate consciousness, mysticism catalyst. Prisoner, prophet, celebrity, highly energized, radical, visionary.

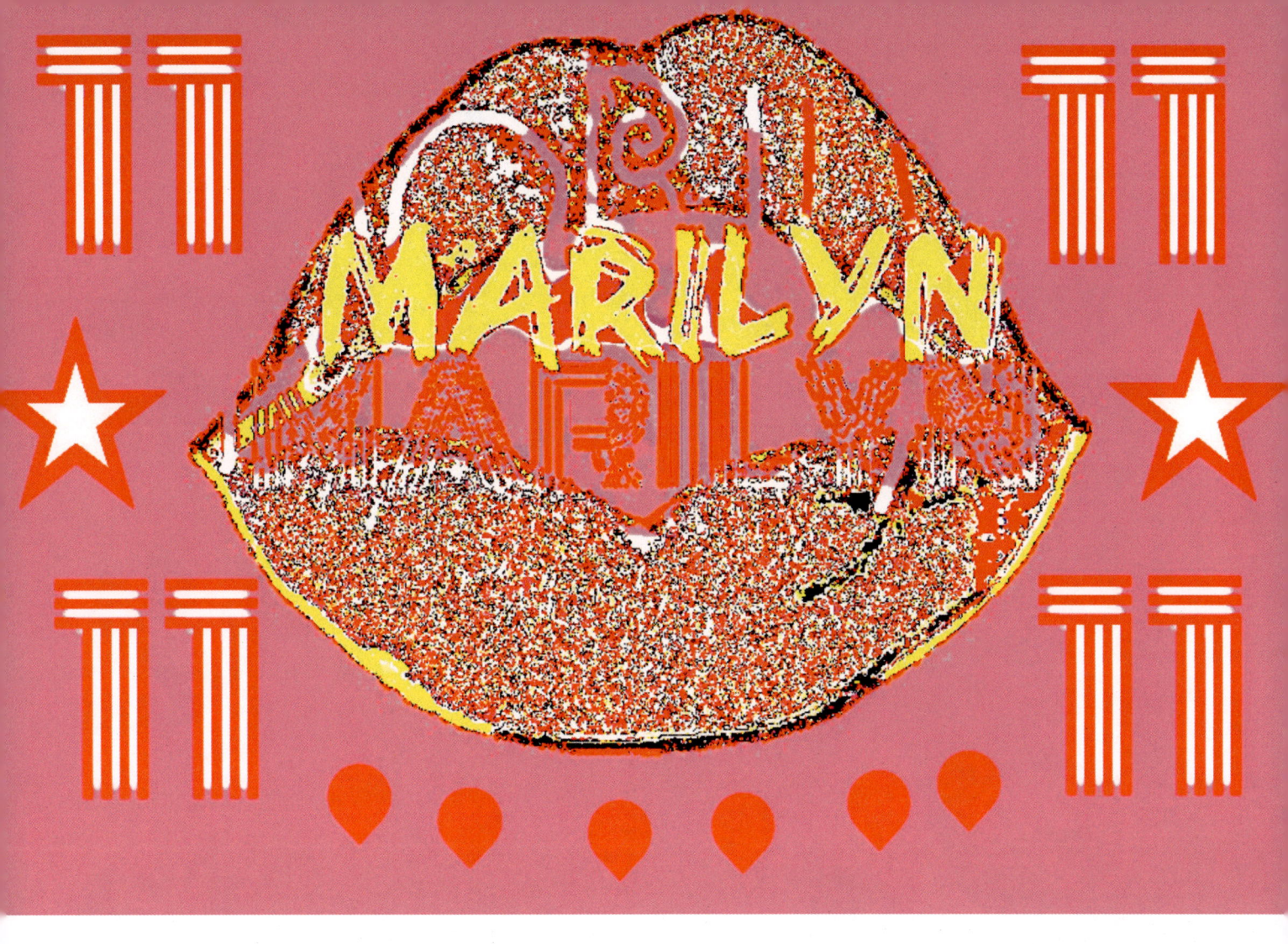

My Duke. You enveloped my heart with a protected shell of thunderous light. You gave me the power to love myself, in my last breath, when I felt lost in the wild. I felt protected in your hands more, than I had ever felt in my life. Like a baby is going backward in time, in a reverse back into his mother's womb. I melted inside of your big father heart. Being carried on your shoulders, while I felt so small, was my biggest blessing.

You were my warm feathers, covering me, in the frozen forest, of my coming end. You had fed me with your honey, and transferred me into a mummy with delight. Like a baby being fed with a warm milk bottle I become the symbol for life after the death. Then I had realized, I had finally met just a few minutes before my end. A pure angel, full with love and light stared at me with your one blue eye. Put down your glass, my duke, my prince, let me kiss you on your lips.

If heaven exists, I had found it at last, one minute before I died in your hands. As long as my body is still warm Let's make love. Ho My Only Duke. Did I tell you I am about to be reborn in the 11 of May 1965? Will you meet me there in the life after life?

Image 144 page 329. Twelve. Model. Painter: Dr. Marilyn Monroe. Photographer: Ofer Frohlich

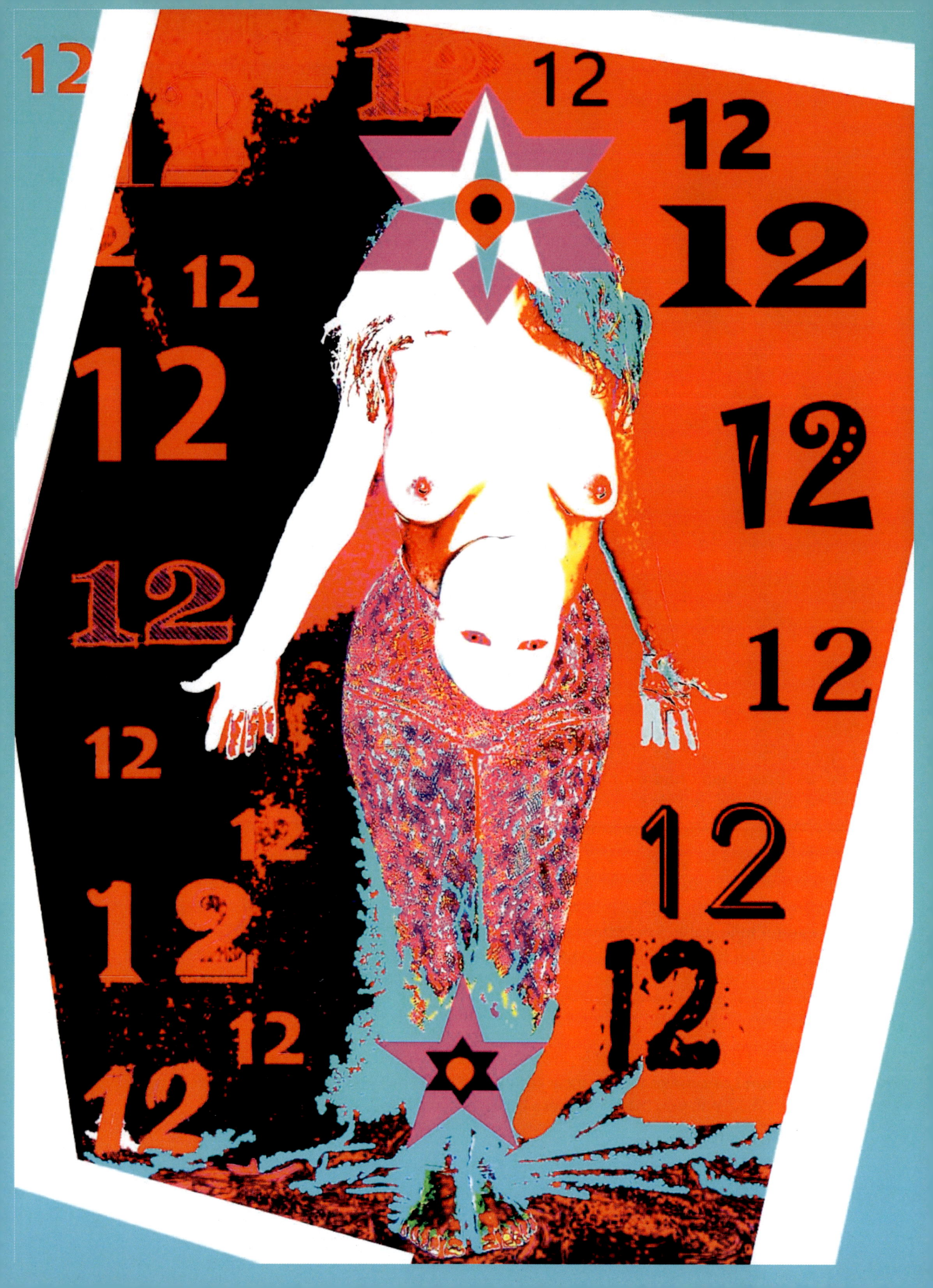
12
12
12
12
12
12
12
12
12
12
12
12
12
12
12
12
12
12

Twelve

Dreams come true - The wishful prince

Mr. President. I am sure, you had asked yourself. How did I get into this situation anyhow? To be captured by this half animal, half human. So. Let me explain what took place ahead to the stage. I was locked in this castle, waiting to become a mummy. This half animal, half man, threatens many people, forced them to take part around my death, signing them on a secrecy contract. Declaring: they understand the importance of keeping my murder in secrets, till the end of their life.

As you probably know, I was fired by the studio from the film "something got to give". But I was ok with that, I desired to achieve making other varieties of roles, in films I will create, in my filming company. The opposite of the superficial, stupid, blonde, sexy character type, I used to carry out. Therefore, I had seen in the studio end of the contract, a sign from God saying to me: I am on the right way, to achieve my goals. To perform my natural talents in acting, and show the world, what I am really made of, as an actress, it was my goal. I knew, my truth talents, is going to be crossed over the scream, as never seen before. I had many scripts in my mind, I wanted to create. One was on my mother's life, I wanted to perform her, I still do. I knew the world had not seen anything yet about my true self, need to.

So, this was the timing, when I was invited for "The weekend with Marilyn, " I was told, they are going to respect my legacy at this weekend, and by using the names of some important people I knew from the industry, they made me believe in their story. They even made me believe, there is going to be present, a true prince," he is your biggest fans Marilyn, he wants to contrive in your motion pictures". What fields my mind was the fact, he can be the cure, for my problematic relations with the Kennedys. If I will derive the title of a princess, next to a respectful prince. John and Bobby Kennedy, will have to apologize for their rudeness attitude toward me, as a sexual toy.

The party which was failing to take place around me, will last around 7 days and nights. It will take place, in one of the most luxurious castles belong to the prince, in France. I will be flying in his private airplane. Only, all this operation, must be kept in secret I was told, the prince asks not to have the press around, he allergic to. Basically, it was something I felt from a very young age, I knew my blood, is coming from a high royal family. The path I drew from being an orphan. With no parents and a stable family, into becoming, one of the biggest glamourous, actress, sex symbol of all times, exhibit the core of souls I belong to, a high class soul. I felt deserved to be honored by a prince, most men, didn't have the courage, to find out, what I am made of. If the prince is from a true royal family, I knew no doubt at all, he will recognize me. One royal soul knows to recognize the other. He will know, how to treat me with the respect I deserve to have. One more benefit adds to it, I will not have to pay with my body and with sex anymore, since men always felt, I need to compensate for my existence, with my physical structure, in order to get appreciation and respect, and in order to serve me the help I need, for my talents to be present. The mysterious prince was only what I needed, to draw out from this cage, cycle, prison, full of brute's rats, simply wants to be feasted with my body, soul, blood and spirit energy, never wished for my wellbeing, or soul, the way I felt I should. Therefore, of course, I approved my participating in this party, but when the prince's soldiers came into my home, to draw me into the plane, I felt strange. They were treated me with not much respect as I should, they were not intolerant, I begin to feel an uncertainty, toward my female instincts, they were too serious, not patient with me. I tried to calm myself down, telling myself, they are just nervous because of me, since I am so famous, they are attempting to show me how serious they are with their work, bringing me safely into the castle, perhaps they are afraid that something will get awry, they took a great deal of responsibility on their shoulders, to bring such a notable name from USA into France, It's a great deal of responsibility. Ok, I said to myself, I have to give faith in them, not to show my suspecting, as my mother used to tell me: Smile Norma Jean, smile. So I did, I smiled. Then I was told, by one of the soldiers in charge: Marilyn, you are about to have nausea along the flight, we need you to take these pills. It will help you to reduce this feeling, please take it before the fly started out, without taking this pill, unfortunately, we will not be able to start the flight. I didn't have any chance, such a big operation is taking place around me, I needed to swallow the little pills to avoid conflicts.

It was the second time I did something against my intuition. I obey them. Right at the moment I did. All my life was taken from me for good, and my "trip to heaven" had begun. Do you see how easy it is, to govern somebody's life. All you necessitate to have is: one good story, a pill, a little reasonable pressure that all. Right afterwards I carried the pill, I begin to feel fragile, dizzy, heavy confused, lazy. Numbly, I didn't lose my conscience, but I lost the power, the will, and the control over my body and mind. This little pill, was the first dose of drugs I will get along my final cut party. Mr. President. I understand, you are about to experience many kinds of disgust and maybe an emotional pain, resonate with my pain along the rest of the book. You may stop reading it now, I am really sorry, I have to participate you with this final cut version. But remember, my surfer is just an exhibition of all the world suffer. I wish a beautiful creation of god as I was, should not be tormented, but If you look at the world we are living in today. It is extremely full with cruelty; I am not the only special one who been every day tormented. I am just trying to wake myself from the dead, in order of bringing a true understanding around children and women's rights. It's my duty toward the human being, to put an end, to all evil methods, which control earth today. Especially toward baby female, and women. We all need to pull together, to fight against it. Marilyn Monroe is not just a beautiful star in the sky, we are all, godly stars in the eyes of the lord.

Number Twelve - 12 meanings

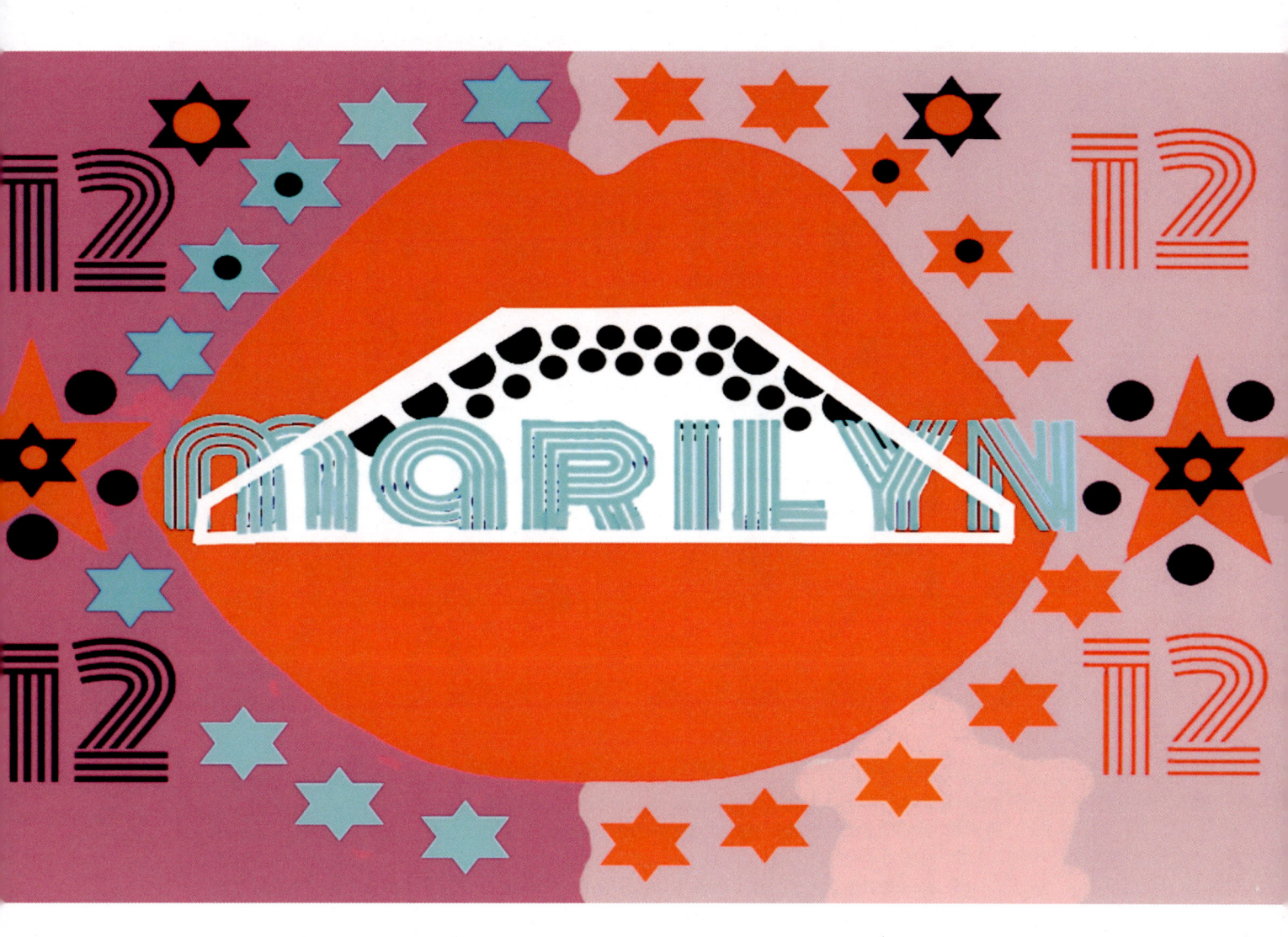

Symbol of cosmic order. Twelve signs in the Zodiac, 12 astrological signs, 12 months in a year. In Judaism, girls become adult toward "Bat Mitzvah" at the age 12. The magnesium Atomic number is 12. Symbol of completed cycle of experience. Achieve knowledge, Wisdom, Spiritual, Intellectual, versatile, energetic, professional, mentally perceptive family conscious, honesty, Laughter, very funny, witty. Inquiring minds, love of people self-insecurities Not shown outside, living a free life, popularity, oozing with charisma. Given freedom, goals achiever. Singers, Versatile, energetic, friendly, individuals, Laughter. Magnetic, vibrating, lovely.

MARILYN MARILYN MARILYN

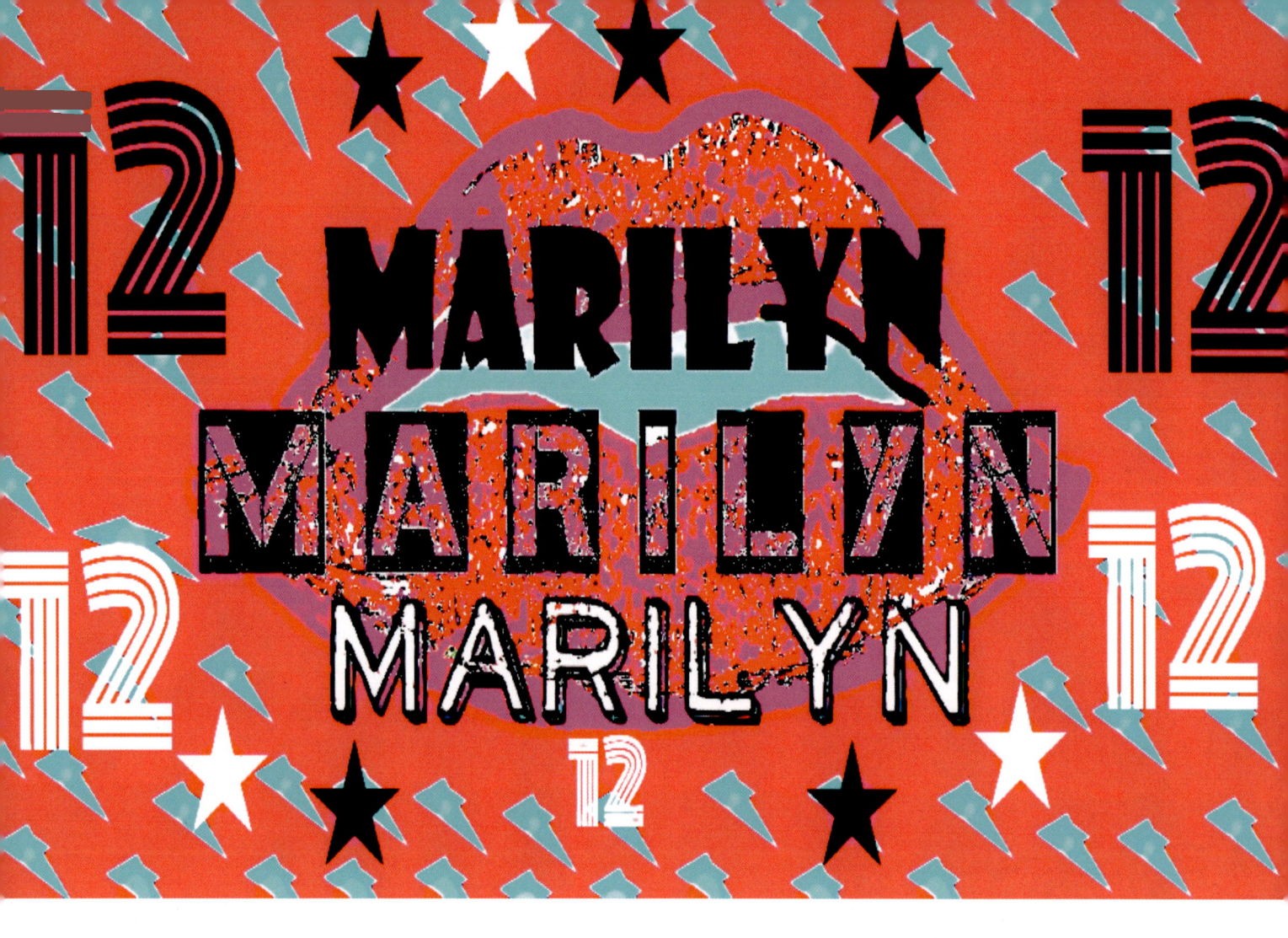

Awakening to the sound of the birds Chirping toward my windows

Seeking for your eyes and their expression of love toward me

Crawling in my bed like a spoiled cat, never want to get out

Wait for the light to get into the room, ascertain you are attending there

Groping with my lips the hem of the pillow.

Tomorrow will be the day Twelve years; I have been wait for.

Tomorrow I will be yours, my holy prince, sent to me direct from the Lord.

You are filling my life with, a deep blue, purple, red, orange, velvet lights.

Once in a lifetime while we will make love.

Two souls embrace with the light.

We will clean the walls of impurity that stuck within our souls.

Wake up from the dead by a loving kiss. After a hundred years of sleeping deep.

Thirteen

The shining star at the black hole in the sky

Mr. president. I was brought into the palace, under the drug effects, I could not suspect something is profoundly wrong, until the point it was too late. The people were wearing a beautiful suit, the music, the ambience, the food, the wine, the dancing atmosphere, everything was just perfect as I expect it to be. A beautiful princess dress was waiting for me, it was a dreamy dress, you had never assured me in such a dress with endless diamonds all over it, yes, pure original diamonds, in any color you can daydream about. I felt as a true princess. I was afraid to sit with this dress; all I could do is dance. I felt my dreams are starting to be fulfilled, heaven is waiting for me. I was not aware witch heaven, it is going to be, the one on earth, or the one up there, I was sent to.

The prince was a decent looking young male. In one of my paintings, I describe in my present life. There is a woman, sitting bare on her knee, she drew a long hair. She got a panicked look inside of her eyes, her facial expression shows, she is horrified by something, next to her standing, a very handsome young prince, looks as a gentleman, with a red parrot next to him. The women look straight into the viewer's eyes, her eyes are full with terror and blood, her lip is open like trying to yell, only her voice in stuck in the middle, it can't run out. She appears under a complete daze, as if she had witnessed the fiend and the angel of death all together. The prince, is in a contrary position to her, he is looking in the other direction, out of the frame of the painting. Looking serene, sure of himself, comfort, quiet. He doesn't express any concern for her misery or suffer. This painting reflecting, what form of heaven, I was facing eventually. From the moment I got to the party, more hidden drugs were added to my glass of wine, made me be a super cooperative, with a completely lacked of ability to refuse in adventure, or anything offered to me. All the men that were present in the main hall, wanted to dance with me; I had never in my life dance with so many men in one endless long evening. Because of the drugs and win, I felt more as a doll swinging, without control on my legs along the floor. The prince gets the honor to have with me the first dance, my head was flying high as a balloon, into the sky, when he holds me tight. I was not aware fully at that time of the evening. I am being shut away inside of this castle, together with 100 men. When I arrived, there were other women present, I watched them dancing. Then gradually, all the other women had disappeared, I was left along with 100 men. I was thinking at first, perhaps they were asked to get dressed for the rest of my party. My brain could not think straight. But who cares, I got the prince all to myself.

Image 145 page 335. Thirteen. Model. Painter: Dr. Marilyn Monroe. Photographer: Ofer Frohlich

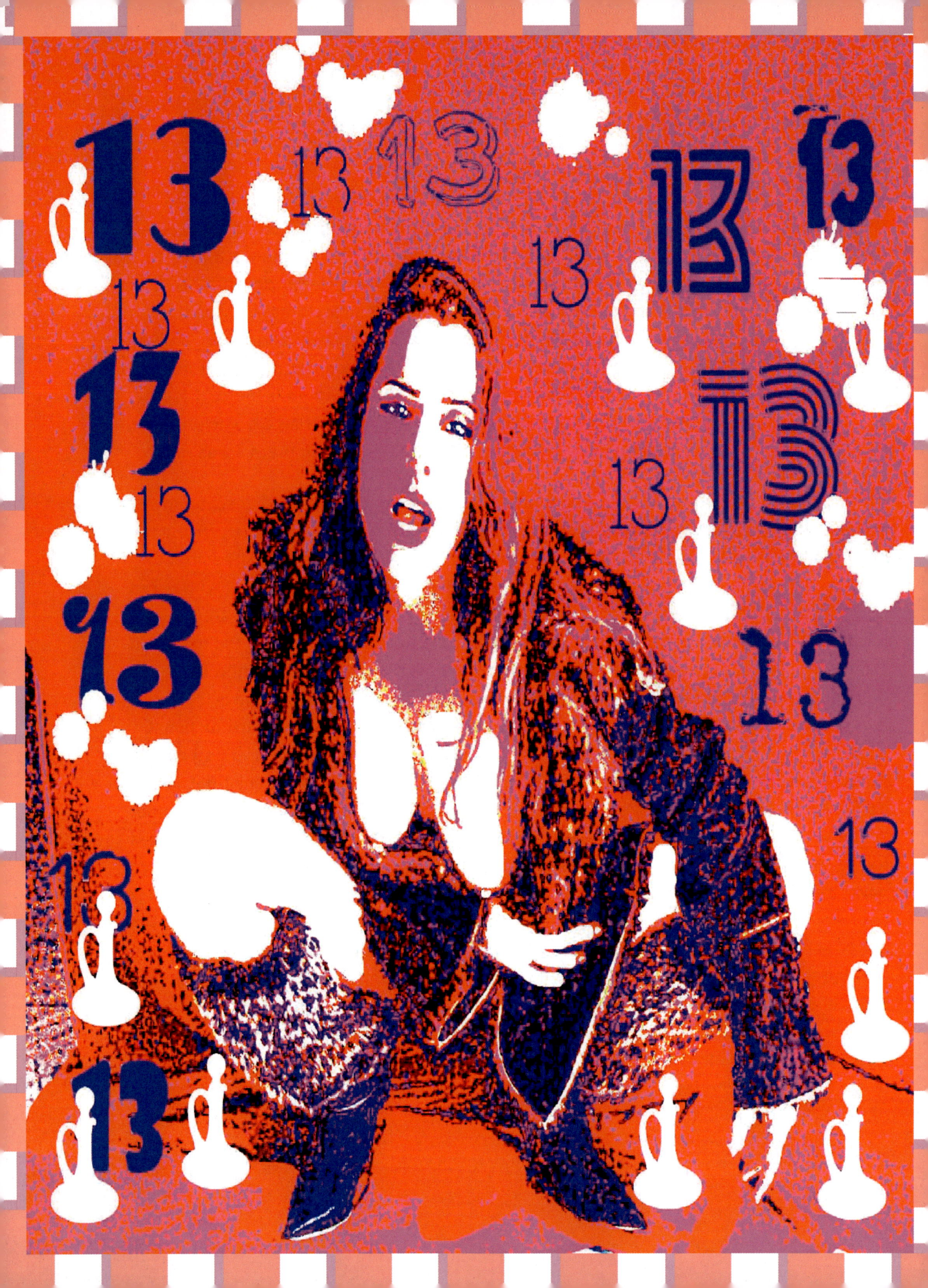
13
13
13
13
13
13
13
13
13
13
13
13
13
13
13
13

The second day came; I didn't remember when I went to sleep. I woke up finding myself to be fully naked, lying along a shining red velvet sheet made of silk, inside of a big auction, around me a hundred of men, sitting and watching me, I attempted to stand upward, only I failed each time I practiced, the overdoses of drugs and alcohol still affect me. The narrow stage I was lying on, was too high I scared to fall from it, I didn't have any control on my legs. Gradually I realized, I am the item for sell. The stage moved slowly in cycles, I tried to come back to myself, in order to hear what are they selling exactly, I was thinking, maybe some kind of jewelry they exhibit on me, as a model. Then I heard, the sale was around the right to have sex with me, I was the item for sell. I start to think, maybe I am participating in a movie scene, I tried to look around, to see if there are any photographers, lightning men, makeup artist, a director, but I found none.

I thought maybe they are all hiding, and when the light will be up I will finally see them. The auction was serious, the atmosphere was quiet, the men didn't move in their chairs too much, they were all wearing a black suit, with a serious look on their faces. Extremely high numbers of cash were throwing in the air, I could not believe this is real, where is the prince? I danced too much the night before, I am sure soon, I will wake up, it must be a dream. Then I heard them selling: 1 the last sex with Marilyn on the red velvet 2. The last oral sex with Marilyn in the bathtub 3. The last anal sex with Marilyn in the doggy style 4. The final dance with Marilyn full nude 5. The last sleeping at night with Marilyn 6. The last kiss with Marilyn, just about I will about to be dead 7. The last meals with Marilyn, food serve on and inside her Marilyn naked body. 8. The last dessert ice cream on Marilyn naked body 9. The last swimming in the pool with Marilyn. A full video film attaches to it.

 They sold as well the right to photograph me.

1. On the cross like Jesus - https://en.wikipedia.org/wiki/Crucifixion_of_Jesus

2. Inside of a cycle. Like in the Leonardo DA Vinci, in the Vitruvian man https://en.wikipedia.org/wiki/Vitruvian_Man

3. Inside of a letter G symbol of God. The letter G being exhibited not once inside of my artistic creation. In one of my paintings, I am making love with a seahorse, while his tail is set in the pattern of the letter G. Almost penetrating the letter V shaped by my legs, there is one more shape, upside down /\. These two V symbols together the Magen David. This symbol is not once being found in my paintings https://en.wikipedia.org/wiki/God

4. Performing with all the letters from A - Z. https://en.wikipedia.org/wiki/English_alphabet

5. Hung up with my head downward, tiny needle will cut each fingertip, I will be moving from side to side above a big white canvas under me. My blood will create this painting.

Number Thirteen - 13 meanings

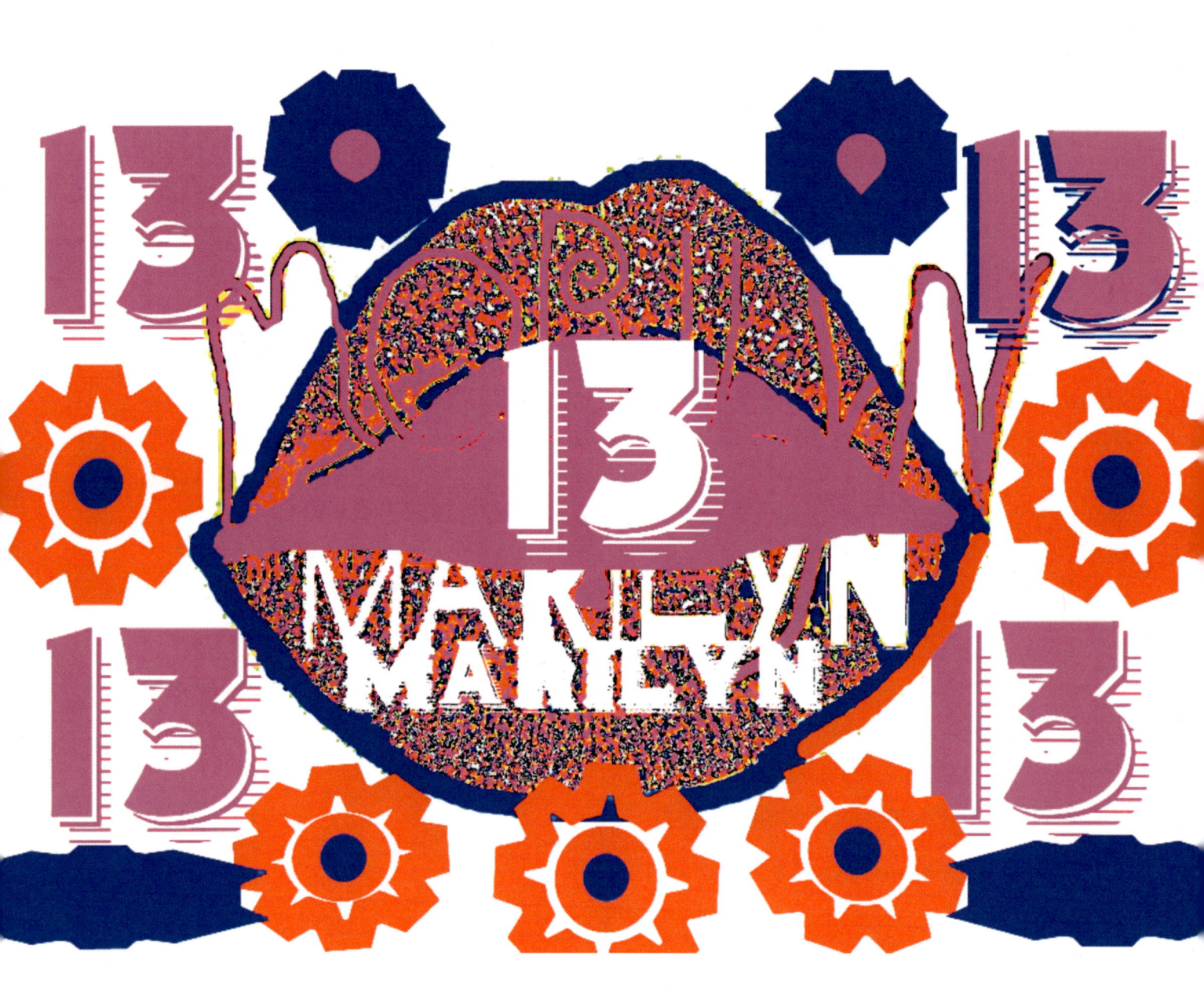

The dragon, Satan, behind all rebellion against God, In Mark 7. Jesus mentions 13 definitions of humanity: adulteries, fornications, evil thoughts, murders Covetousness thefts, wickedness, licentiousness, guile, blasphemy, foolishness, pride, an evil eye Ishmael Abraham, son, were circumcised, cut off of the foreskin of a penis, when he was 13. A devilish number, a blessing promise number. The 13th card inside of the Tarot cards is of a skeleton. In the United States, the first national flag had 13 stars, on the green side of the dollar bill 13 steps in the pyramid of the Great Seal. Star Sirius longitude 13°. The Indian Pantheon got 13 Buddha's. The ancient Mexicans number of 13 snake Gods. The English 13th letter is Mam. Mother. Marilyn Monroe. MM. Maria Magdalena. Mary Jesus mother.

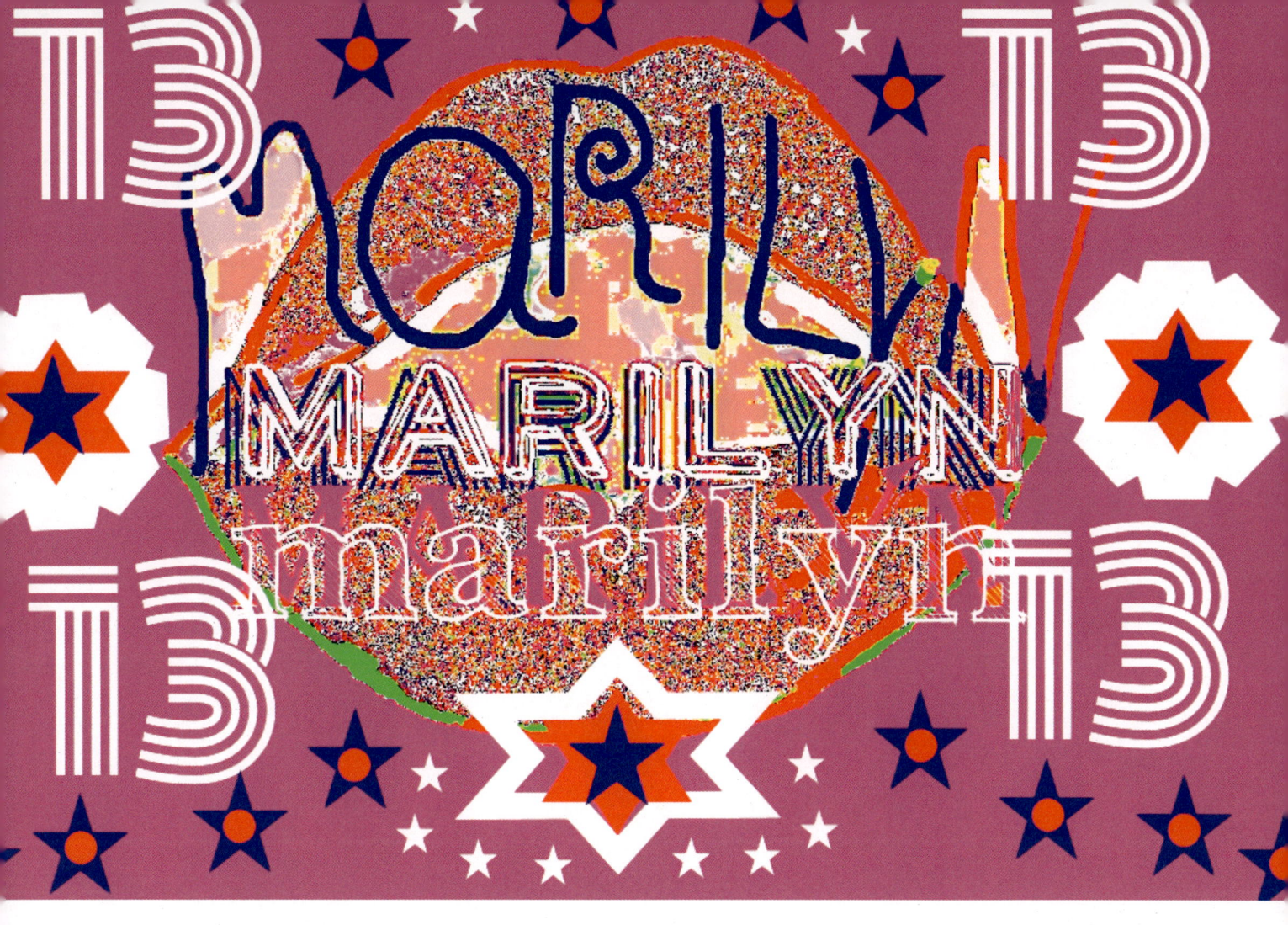

When the train of your life is a runaway. Do not stop to wait for me on the side way. Just show me the way back to the grave I was taken out of. The grave I was buried inside secretly, In the middle of the night. From my grave I will make a jump with my eyes wide open. Right into your brandy bottle, pretend life had never been better. I will teach you to drink your wine mix with my blood. Break free Thirteen time, from all the spells you made around me from to the present life

Then I will watch you walking in cycles, around your poor existence. Give you a little youth directly from my veins. Feed you with a new red energetic blood full with Chi. It will smooth back all the wrinkles that had gathered on your face. It will give you the power you need to fight for your life once more. Like a unicorn. Then I will jump on you and we will make a ride. Up and down from the bottom of the Godly bottle. We will ride right into the Godly nest and his heavenly warmth womb.

Image 146 page 339. Fourteen. Model. Painter: Dr. Marilyn Monroe. Photographer: Ofer Frohlich

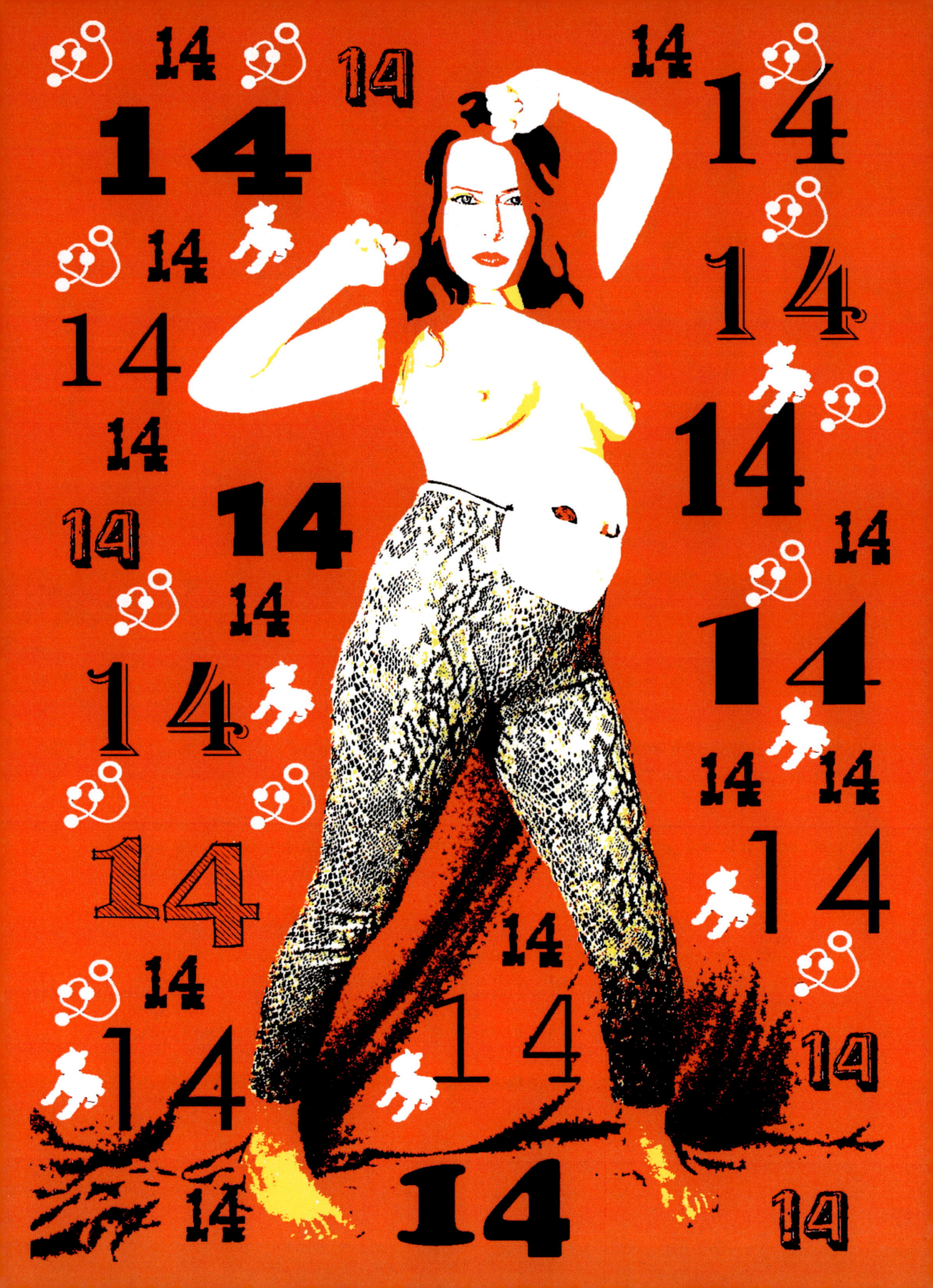

Fourteen

Marilyn last supper

Mr. President. This is the list of the last prices, which my body pieces were traded, inside of the auction: My brain was sold separated from the remainder of my body for 1500.000.000$. I am not sure if they meant to prune it out from my physical structure, present it as a sculpture mummy by itself. Or all together with the rest of my body, since the prince asked to buy it, as the Duke told me. He offered 50 million $ to get my head back into its place, or basically, to leave it there. And not separated it from the rest of my body. It definitely shows the passion he had toward me.

It is warming my heart knowing, how dear I was for the prince. I found out afterwards, he could not take me as his wife, because of his family members. They didn't allow him to have me. Therefore, he has done everything in his power, to have all of me as one piece of art, as a sculpture mummy. Ho. My prince charming, you are a truth heart breaker. It will be interesting to reveal, his secret museum under the ground in Paris, near the Louver, in France, to found out, how I am presented. Do you think, he left me full naked mummy?

Regard my inside diamond brain, it was sold separately for 190.000.000$. My Heart was sold for approximately 90.000.000$, My Liver was sold for 85.000.000$. Mr. president, I am sorry. This is not enough, I expected to a higher price on my head. At least 500.000.000$. 190.000.000$ is not what I assessment and value of my head. They should have charged for it more, much more. Let's test what this group of animal boys paid for the rest of my body parts: My Spain was sold for 80.000.000$, my colony sold for 60.000.000$. My Womb was sold for 55.000.000$.

My Kidney sold for 45.000.000$ each. My lung was sold for 40.000.000 $ each, my pancreas was sold for 35.000.000$. My duodenal was a sold for 30.000.000$. My diaphragm was sold for 29.000.000$. My small intestine was sold for 28.000.000$. My Spleen was sold vertebra for 25.000.000$ each. The tissues around my organs. Which usually being thrown, they were sold for the purpose of cooking with it the final supper from my soft flesh, for approximately of 80.000.000$. They have eaten at the last supper with Marilyn.

Finally, my tissues were supposed to be delivered as an art ceremony, a recreation of the last supper with Jesus. My blood, were about to be turned over to the people to drink, almost all my Death procedure was similar to Jesus, with one huge difference. Jesus death was displayed outside, where everybody could watch him suffer, witness his last agony. In my case it was secretively hidden from the public eye.

Image 147 page 341. Fourteen. Model. Painter: Dr. Marilyn Monroe. Photographer: Ofer Frohlich

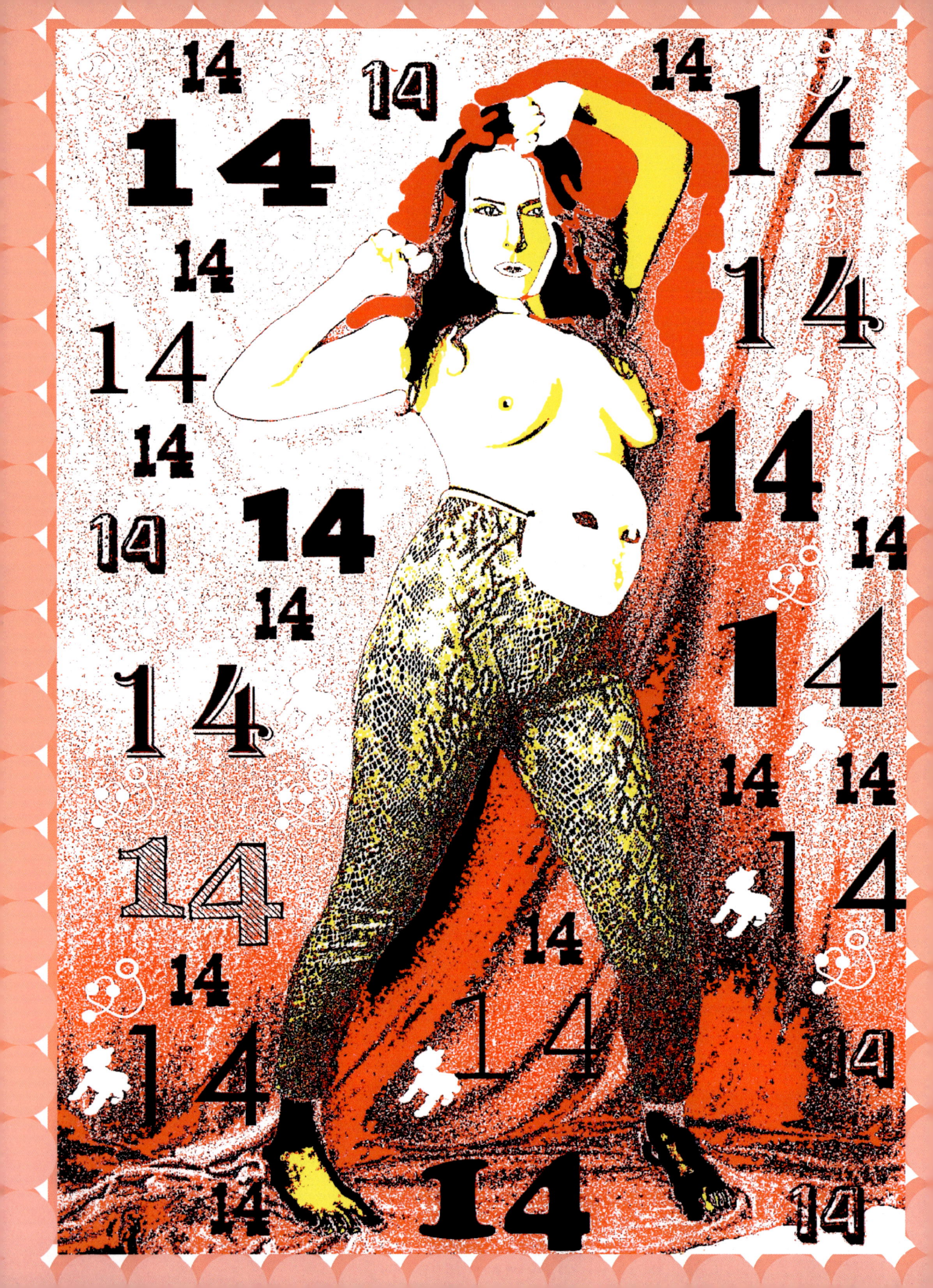

Did you know Mr. president, God. He had never witnessed in me just a sex symbol, like your man does. No, he didn't, God. Looks straight into my eyes and into my soul, since he creates me full with his brightness and internal illumination, full with his cognition, full with his vibration of respect for any living being, and for life, He sees my purity beyond any sex symbol titles. God sees in me the medicine, and the cure, and "the rescue remedy" he made specially for you, for all humankind. I was born to be your medicine for your wounded souls. Apparently, I am as well, God medicine and cure. For his own pains, all the pain and headache humanity is causing him, killing one another, Killing his best creation as they did with me, killing his best creations. God is crying, and I am wiping his tears. Theses is why he wanted me to come back, in order to make a worldly overall change, in the conscience of the world, around his creation, to teach humanity to respect his creations. It will be a metrical for him, and a cure for him, if I will manage to come back fully to life.

God requires me to get an overall peace to the Earth, to give up any motivation whatsoever behind any sort of murder and violent death, as human is used to take in their hands, another human life so easily. Without considering thinking twice, about the Lord creatively, he invents the human race. Which is executed. I am Marilyn, just one sample of the millions that had been killed over the years, from the time humans get the privilege to have life, by the Lord. The creator of all humans. All the killings made around the world each moment, are against the Lord soul and his will. Therefore, he made me, as his remedy, to keep him smile even time after a cruelty, death appears to make his day shine. Which this is what I am doing. Unless I did, he would be crying all day long.

When I came back to the lord, in 4 - 5 August 1962, God didn't require me to run down once more. He was exceedingly disappointed with the way humanity treat me as Marilyn Monroe. He told me: Marilyn, if you are going there once more, you need to know, all human is going to kick your ass in any possible way. If you go there once more, especially if you will exhibit yourself as the coming back Marilyn Monroe, humanity is going to overly freak out. They don't recognize my power to bring you back to life, they are so limited in their ability to see the soul of the matter, they will not go to recognize you, since you are not going to look exactly the same. They will call you crazy, nut.

They are going to hate you, especially all the fans you had left behind as Marilyn, this fan is feeling a bond, an ownership of your body and soul. They compete with one another who owns more of you. While me and you know they own nothing at all, they even don't know your soul as should, if they do, I could transfer you back to be a monkey, and they could still recognize you under any outside shape or form, if they could really see your soul, but they can't, they are blind This is the main reason, why they will hate you like you are Hitler. Actually, they are going to hate you much more than Hitler, they will think you are the devil, the Daughter of the Devil believes you are coming into being a holocaust.

Image 148 page 343. Fourteen. Model. Painter: Dr. Marilyn Monroe. Photographer: Ofer Frohlich

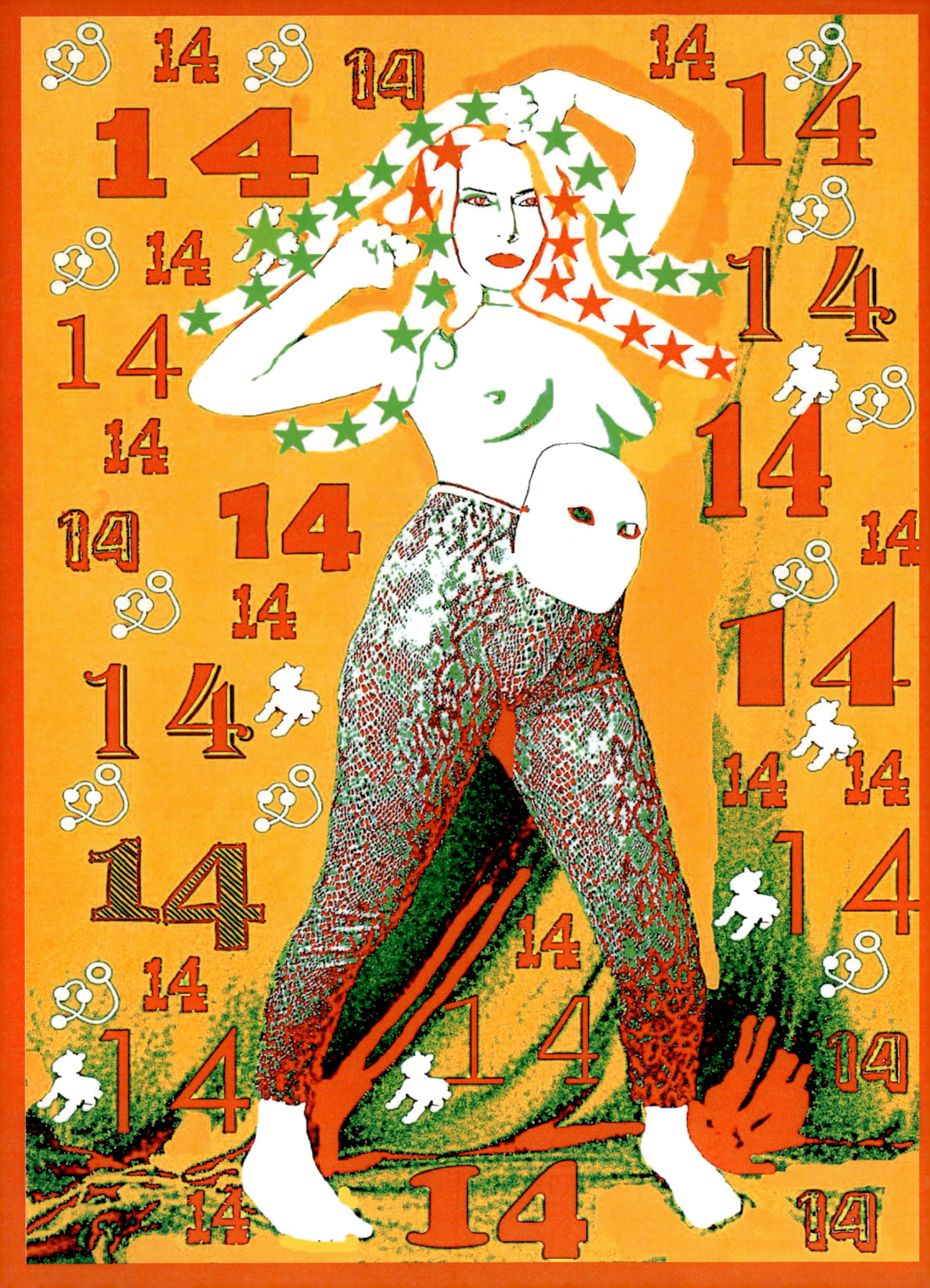

But Marilyn, if you insist to go down there, back into hell, I will give you are the support you need to overcome any obstacle. In order to bring back a full justice for your soul, free yourself from any prejudice. Then I will help you, it will make me happy, to see my most lovable daughter wins against all odd, since I created you in that fashion, it will warm my heart. Mr. president. The last supper with and of Marilyn Monroe is what it was. http://en.wikipedia.org/wiki/Last_Supper – it was a justified murder. The human witch operated it got a good excuse behind their activities, they supposed they helps "me" cleanse my soul, help "me" purify myself. As mentioned: My last supper contains drinking wine made by my blood, food produced by my internal tissue, along the wall of the big Banquet feast, they hang a great signal, saying: "Lets Purify Marilyn Monroe soul"

They truly believed, their soul will be elevated by God, because they served me to " pure myself ". You know what's really funny? They did a great job, yes they did, help me purify my soul, they helped me feel so tormented, this torment pushed me to start work harder, on my escape, from all the kinds of prison I gain along the way, from the first day God created me, along all the lifetimes I had, which made me become more and more locked inside, not being able to express my soul.

You think. I am straining to overcompensate with my attitude, on the not digestible cruel, inhuman murder I went to. I understand what you mean, since no human can tolerate the fact, his murder is for the best for him, as well as myself, I am completely against any kind of violation of the human right to live with respect. Side by side to it, I am trying to consider the Lord point of sight, why did the God manage to feed the human hand, the power to bump off one another? Why? He could prevent it all together from the beginning. Prevent all together from millions of people to get killed, in any fashionable way by one another.

God possessed the ability to execute anything, he could simply make human with no ability in their brain cells, of thinking about the need to murder some other human. He could program us as such. Why didn't he do it then? I am trying to catch the good side of it, to make it painless. I had investigated it deeper, from the Lord point of perspective, what I had found out, is against what I wanted, and or you wish to hear. Obviously, my murder was the solitary path, god could change me into the correct level of infinity I deserve to be in, into the kingdom of souls, the royal family's souls I belong. Unfortunately, without pain there is no game.

These half human, half beasts, up until today. They are keeping part of my physique in the frozen breeze, applying it every year. Like in the sacrament, sharing tiny pieces of my flesh, inside of a special celebration around each 5 of August. I have to consult with you around this point. Do you believe, eating me and recreating the last supper with my flesh and blood, was anything to do with my changing over into a Judaism, before I got married to Arthur Miller?

Number Fourteen - 14 meanings

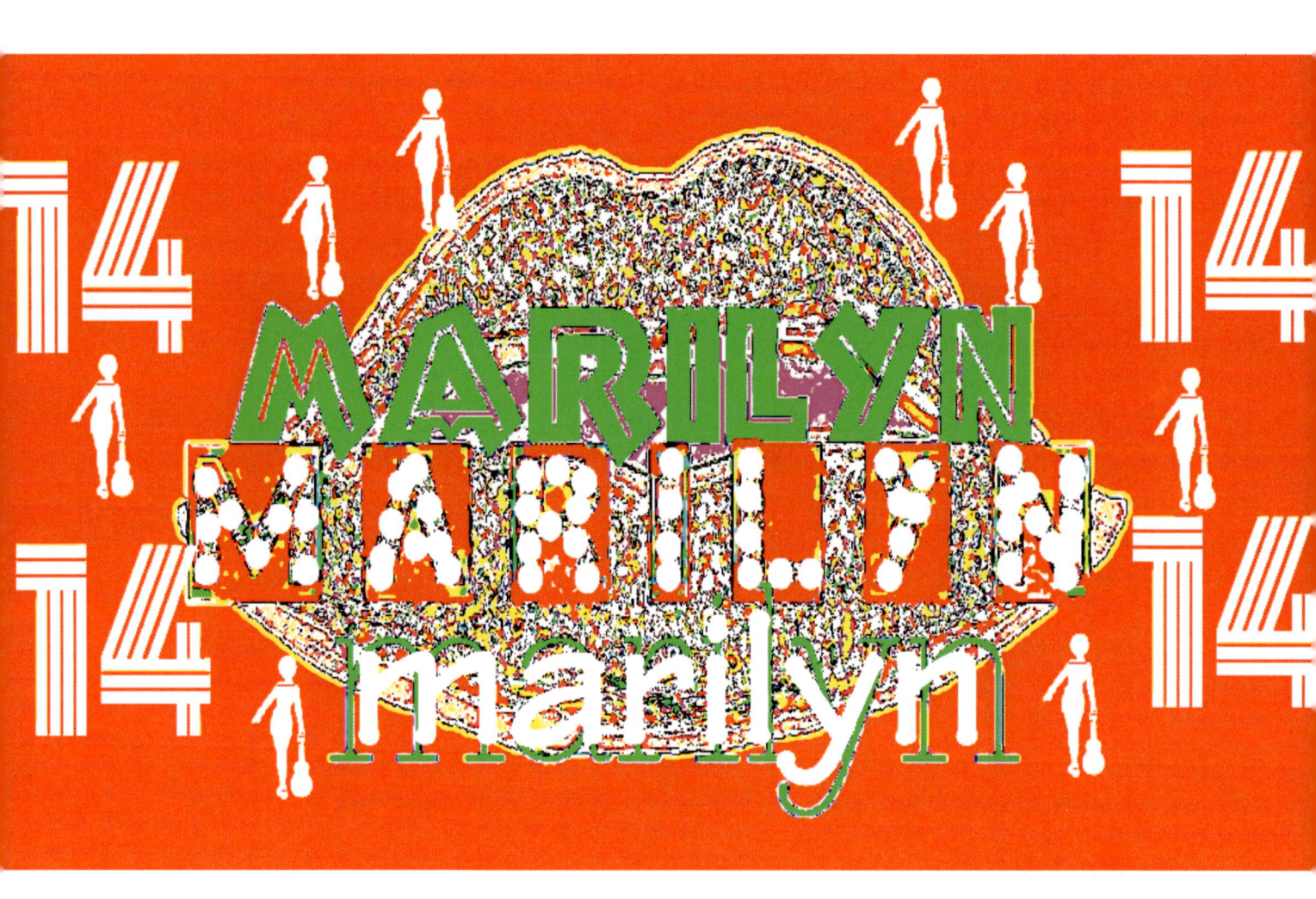

Deliverance or salvation. On the 14th day of the first month. Jesus Christ, God manifested in the flesh, a karmic number, learning independence, unity justice. Harmony, prudence. Experience. Chaos, a progressive change strong influence on people, single-minded businesses, ventures, open, innovative change. A constant challenge, become bored capacity for love, socially popular. Fearless reckless, question, seek high-risk, creativity, wisdom, a roller coaster. Headstrong. Methodical, prodigal pessimist. Ambition, money, greed. Leadership, initiative, Money-orientate, not sincere. Very, Polite. diplomat.

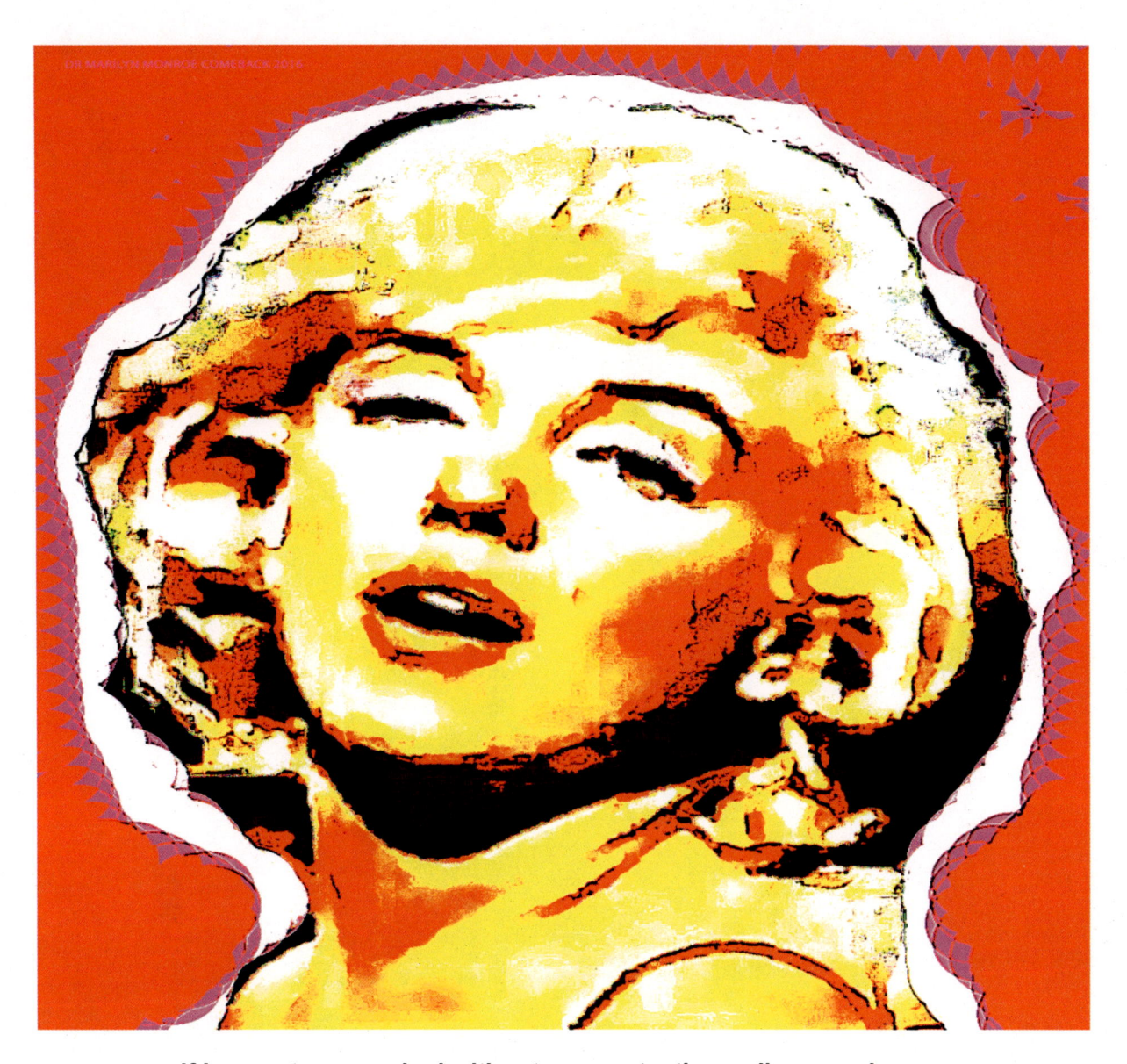

If I come to you naked without any protective walls around me

Will you tie me to your sinking ship's ropes. Engage me in your roller coaster ride.

Made me start engine your soul Fourteen time in a row. Let you head dive inside of the interminable space. Fast and hard until you will finish your drive

Than. You will come hungry and barefoot back to me. Like a little child

Needing to suck from his mother breast. You will run along endless deserts

Finally, when you will arrive trying to catch me with your hands

You will witness how my body being diffused, into the rocks and ground.

How my soul had lifted under a giant wave, high above the sky.

Hiding in between the cloud. As a flag of sanity, at the bottom of the endless stars

Image 149 page 347. Fifteen. Model. Painter: Dr. Marilyn Monroe. Photographer: Ofer Frohlich

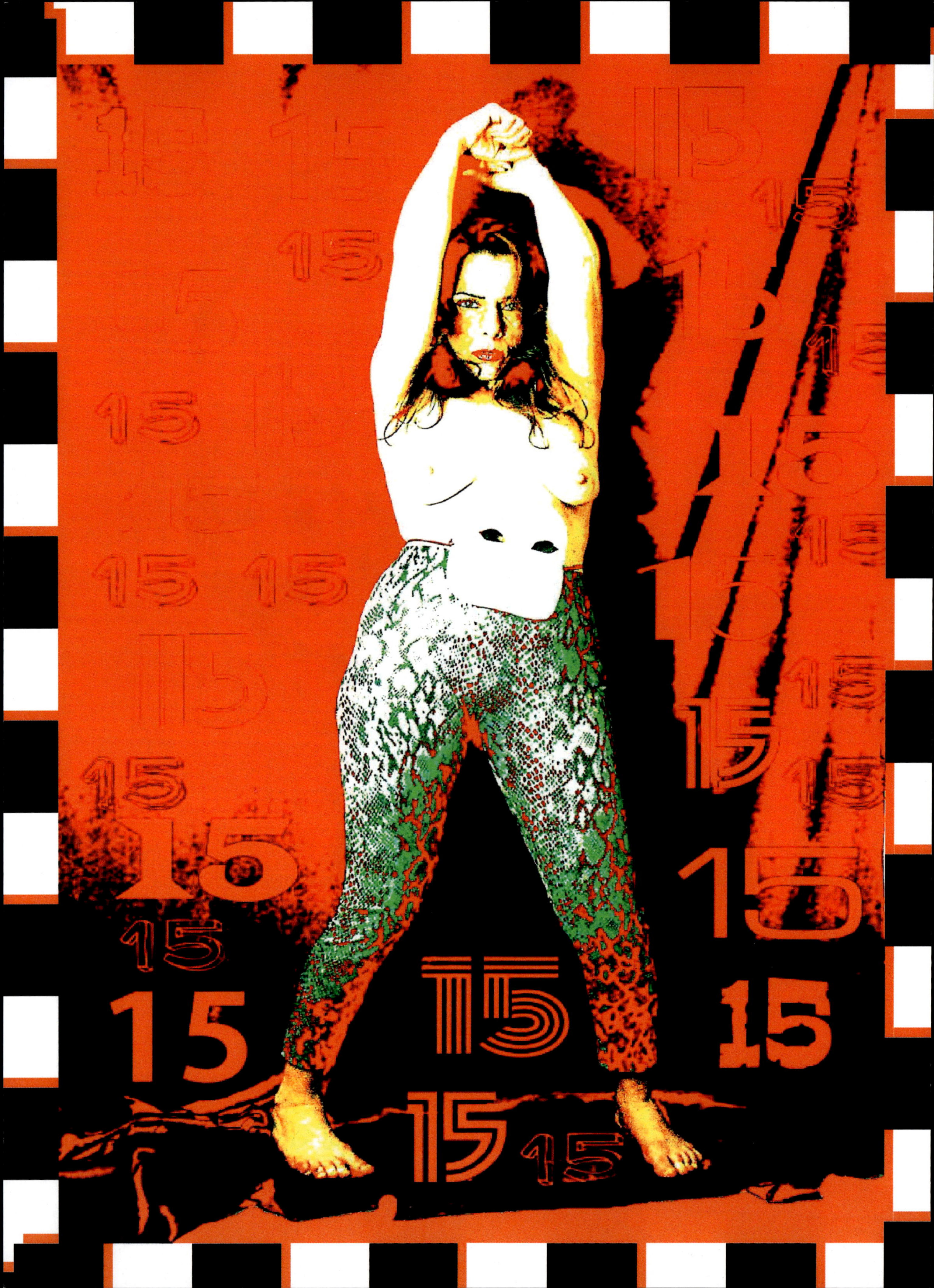
15
15
15
15
15
15
15
15
15
15
15
15

Fifteen

Electra complex – and the red pelages

Mr. President. My wounds around the father figure, had never cured, I was looking for a father to take care of me, protect me, give his hand, adopt me, prove unconditional love toward me. This sort of the "Red Riding Hood" state of mind, I believe, had finally led to that destruction. My "Electra unsolved complex" problem, had cut through space and time, ultimately as any other soul character I had within me, it as well made a big jump together with me, landing inside of the present. Even my extremely good father, Moses could not help me cure this gate in time. No one could, I was going after my own past life tail helplessly, trying to get the missing component of my missing past life father, I missed back there in the channel of my past life. I jumped on any mature adult males, which was imitating the male parent figure, exhibit to me "as if" a true unconditional love toward me.

Sometimes I had found myself with men at the age of my grandpas. It just prof my research for the father figure of my past life, was locked forever deep inside my sub conscience with no way out. A precious moment, frozen forever in time. The amount of years, these men in the present were around the age 55 - 68, exhibiting my soul need to make a connection, with a man at the same age of time, as was my missing father I left behind, at the time of my death in 1962. Through this man I was trying to send a message to my father, which was locked inside of a vacuum hole in my past.

This emptiness inside of my soul, which needed and try to fulfill itself over and over by endless older men, was an outcome to the fact, I had never managed to meet my truth father, the one who made me with my mother, Gladys, this dream I had in my past to one day be able to finally know for sure and meet my own father drained me back in time at the present, with no escape. There was nothing I could fulfil this hole of conscience with, it's haunted me into the present, didn't leave me the ability to live and enjoy in the present, as I should, with my present life father Moses.

http://en.wikipedia.org/wiki/Little_Red_Riding_Hood.

http://en.wikipedia.org/wiki/Electra_complex

I start portrait myself again in full nude from the age 14. Performing who I am transferring into this present. For me there was no past, death, and present. Simply, one lineage of life that has no beginning and no end. The nude photography, paintings, video. People believed I am doing it, for bringing an extra "attention".

But for me my nude soul, is the one I exhibit not my body, my body is but a chariot inside of, my soul can drive and be present on earth. My godly core, don't ask of me to hide behind my flesh, it is as well, not a sin, to reveal what the creator creates inside of me. The divine Creator fulfills me toward his vitality. If there was a sex element in my life inside of my art, it the sexuality God add into this creation. Within God eyes, the sexuality he purred inside of me. The godly passionate he spills inside of me, was in his and my eyes never a symbol of gender of a lewd thought around sex, the way people translate it. I have not witnessed myself as a sex symbol. To be a sex symbol is really trivial. I got a such a big brain, whatever component of my art created in my past, as easily in the present, it was always being governed by my brain.

The godly light, was spilled inside of me, this is how God shin his light spirit energy, toward arts. I surrender myself to the master of the universe, his spirit hovering me, hugging me, knows me intimately. I never needed to hide from him. What you are witnessing toward my art, Is the procedure of making love with God. This is the reason why, the only clothes I ask to lay in front of the Lord, while we are making love, is my soul envelop inside of a nude body. The dress I wear for the John Kenney birthday party, meant to give John, for his birthday party, the ability to feel, as if he can touch me toward this dress, in front of all. It was a way to make love with John, in front of the universe. I wanted everybody to witness how deeply in love we are. How much we vibrate like "one-coin soul" when we are near. Buy this dress, I desired to have him thinking about how it will be holding our marriage ceremony. It was why I pick the color silver, for this dress.

Today I know. Some of my nude exposers, gave one more hidden motivations, to kill me. Taking into consideration the fact, at the 1 in July 1956 I become Jewish, while being Jewish, I made the first exposure of nudity in the film "something got to give". Non female actress before made such a nude scene inside of a cinema, many men were present on the set, some were Jewish. I was fully naked it against their religion. I am not trying to point out, Jewish people were after my death. But to show off the fact many men, felt I was breaking many roles. If I can break so easily so many roles as a Jew girl, they thought they can break more rules, by easily governed their animal desires.

While all what I was doing is exhibiting art, breaking the border lines inside of the art world, I tried to be the best actress I could, to earn like Elizabeth Taylor. Back in 1949, when I did my first nude with the photographer, Tom Kelley Sir, performed later inside of the playboy magazine. There was a big chaos around it. Human is respecting the fact "David the kind" sculpture is being present in full nude on the street, his sexual organs are fully disclosed, have you ever heard anyone in the world complaining, about the fact: this sculpture exhibit in public places, where children are passing. David sculpture produced it 1501-1504. Today, 511 years later, humanity reaction is more immature toward a nude art.
https://en.wikipedia.org/wiki/David_(Michelangelo)

Number Fifteen - 15 meanings

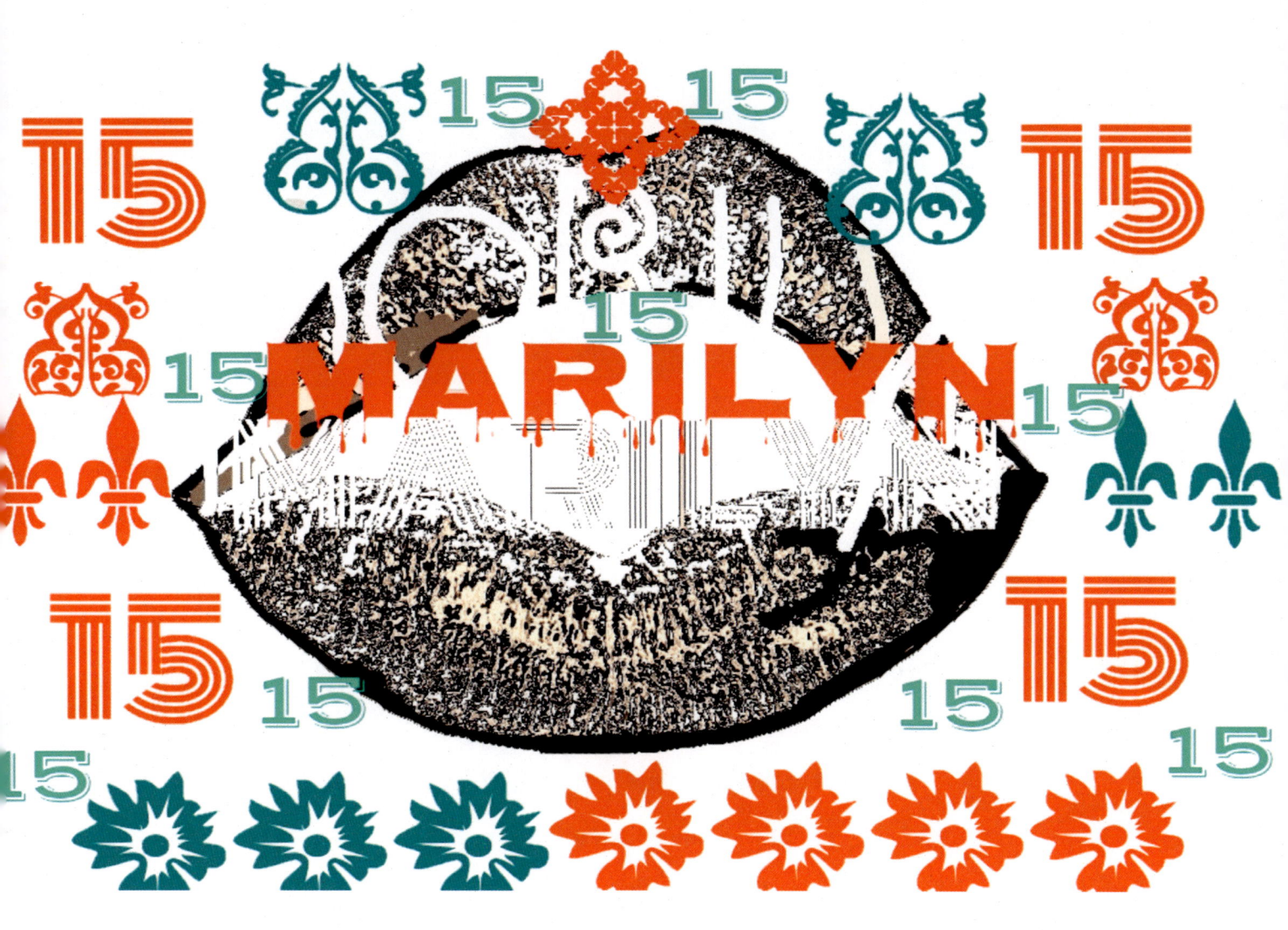

Jesus body placed in a Tomb as the sun was setting to Nisan 15. Private life. Security settled family, need of affection, independent, quite rebellious, vulnerable soft, loving loyal. Faithful, caring, the phosphorus atomic number is 15. May 15th - International Day of Families Tarot 15 is the card of the Devil - failure or reduction. Abraham Lincoln died February 15, 1865. Julius Caesar murdered on March 15. Curious, involuntary leader, subordinate to the family, harmony, home Vibration. Responsibility, healing, domestic activity. Beauty, comfort. Adventure, Determined too express. Self-sacrifice, extremely need for protection. Cause of being associated

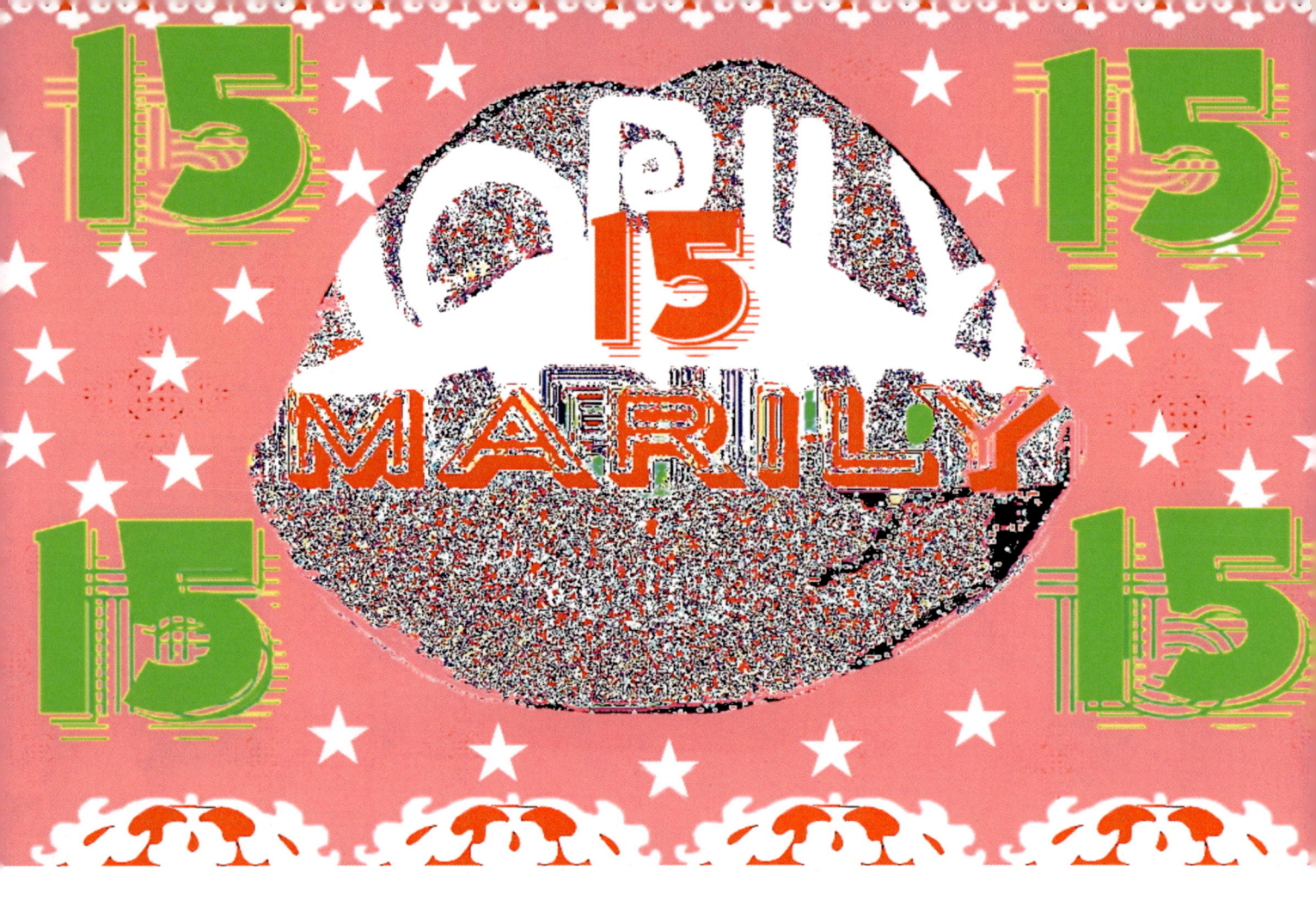

My desire for you covered with morning fog.

When I am rolling in bed, all I can think of is when will You come back.

You penetrate with your spirit into the deepest holes inside of my soul.

Where I could not escape, from hugging you deep within.

I was enveloped myself inside of

A cloud, when you were late to arrive.

Leaving my shadows, to fall into the empty spaces of my hollow heart.

Inside my heart, the lessons of life, carried me away from you.

But could never take my memory far. We missed the track, nothing proves you left

Except the floating bridge over the Islands. There, we transparent into birds

dancing Inside of the wide sky. Like two lost astronaut floating forever in space.

We passed on our boundaries away, flight high, where no one will be able to found us

Into the Fifteen hidden dimension of the light

Sixteen

The Ten Commands

Mr. President. It is a good timing to consider these Ten Godly Commands. I don't mind to give an example; regard good or bad things I had done in my life which are against the Ten Commence. I know, disobedient to this Ten Commandments, is destructive. I consider this commandment, are not just truth in the Jewish religious, they are a universal rule. Side by side to it, any rules had its exceptions. For example, if you look at the ten commands, the biggest crime I had done was to flirt with married men in both lives, in my heart, I don't think people should hold their marriage, if there is no truth love in it. But, if they are having children, they should try to work on their love connection. I worked and performed in a single party's, of couples before they are getting married. And teach them all the secret of love, and passion. In order to know how to keep the fire of love.

I am against betraying, even, I was not once the cause for such. What I mean is, a secret love affair is wrong, it should not be made out under the spine of your partner, if the partner doesn't know, he cannot protect himself or the marriage. The best is, to get married with your soul mate, which completes you, not antagonist to you, a true passion and a serious lovemaking are important. People need to beware of the reasons, what made them choose one another as a partner for a lifetime. I do believe men could have 2 wives, and females could have 2 husbands. If one of the partners is finding himself in love with another person, instead of breaking all the structure of the family, they should become wider. Besides that, I believe in the Ten commence. This rule is unguarded by humanity, this is why the universe is under a chaotic, Schizophrenia state of mind. And the most beautiful creatures in the universe being murdered as I did.

http://en.wikipedia.org/wiki/Ten_Commandments

- I am the LORD thy God
- Thou shalt have no other gods
- No graven images or likenesses
- Not take the LORD's name in vain
- Remember the Sabbath day
- Honor thy father and thy mother
- Thou shalt not kill
- Thou shalt not commit adultery
- Thou shalt not steal
- Thou shalt not bear false witness
- Thou shalt not covet

Image 150 page 353. Sixteen. Model. Painter: Dr. Marilyn Monroe. Photographer: Ofer Frohlich

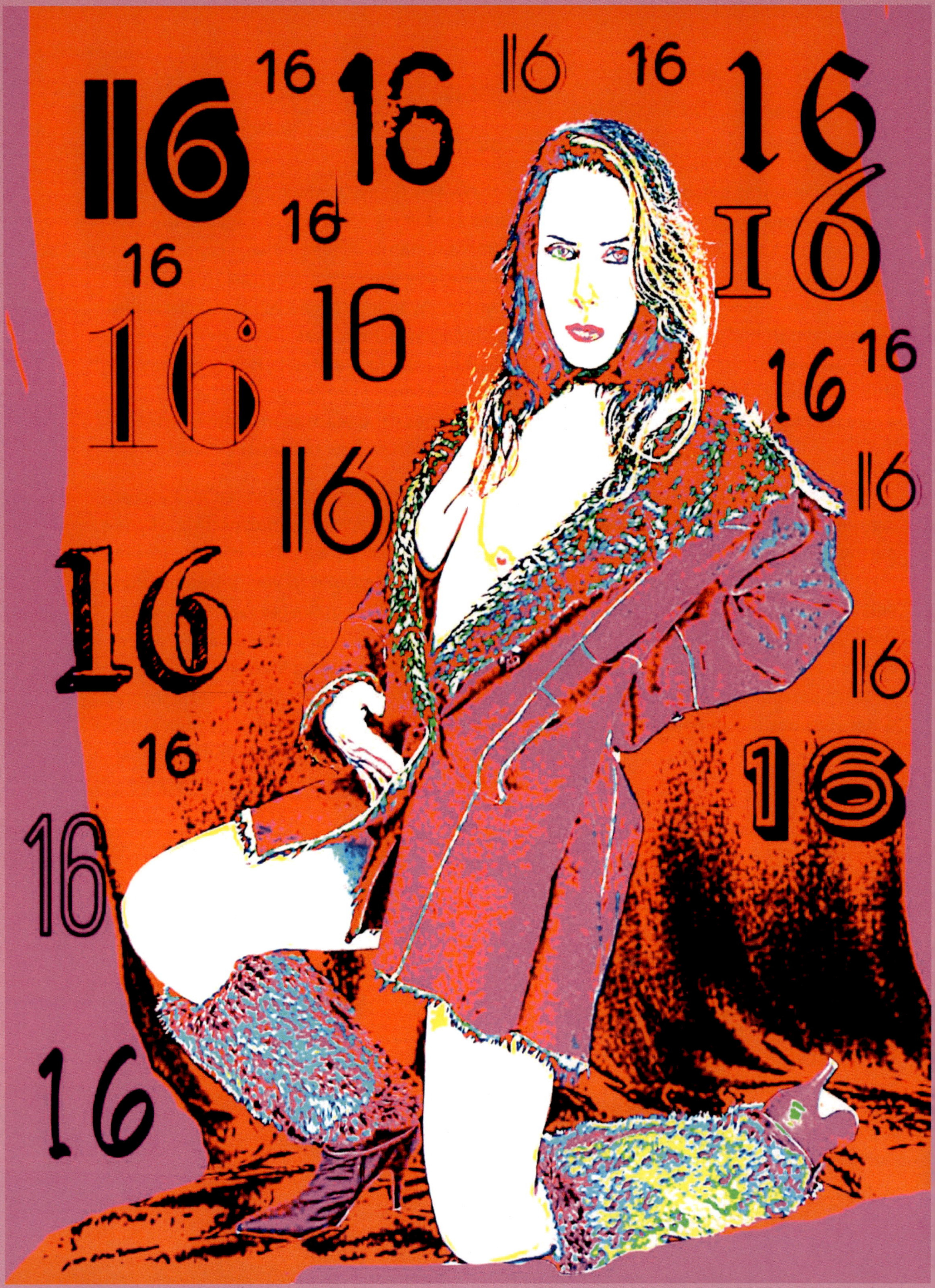
16
16
16
16
16
16
16
16
16
16
16
16
16
16
16
16
16
16
16
16
16

Number Sixteen - 16 meanings

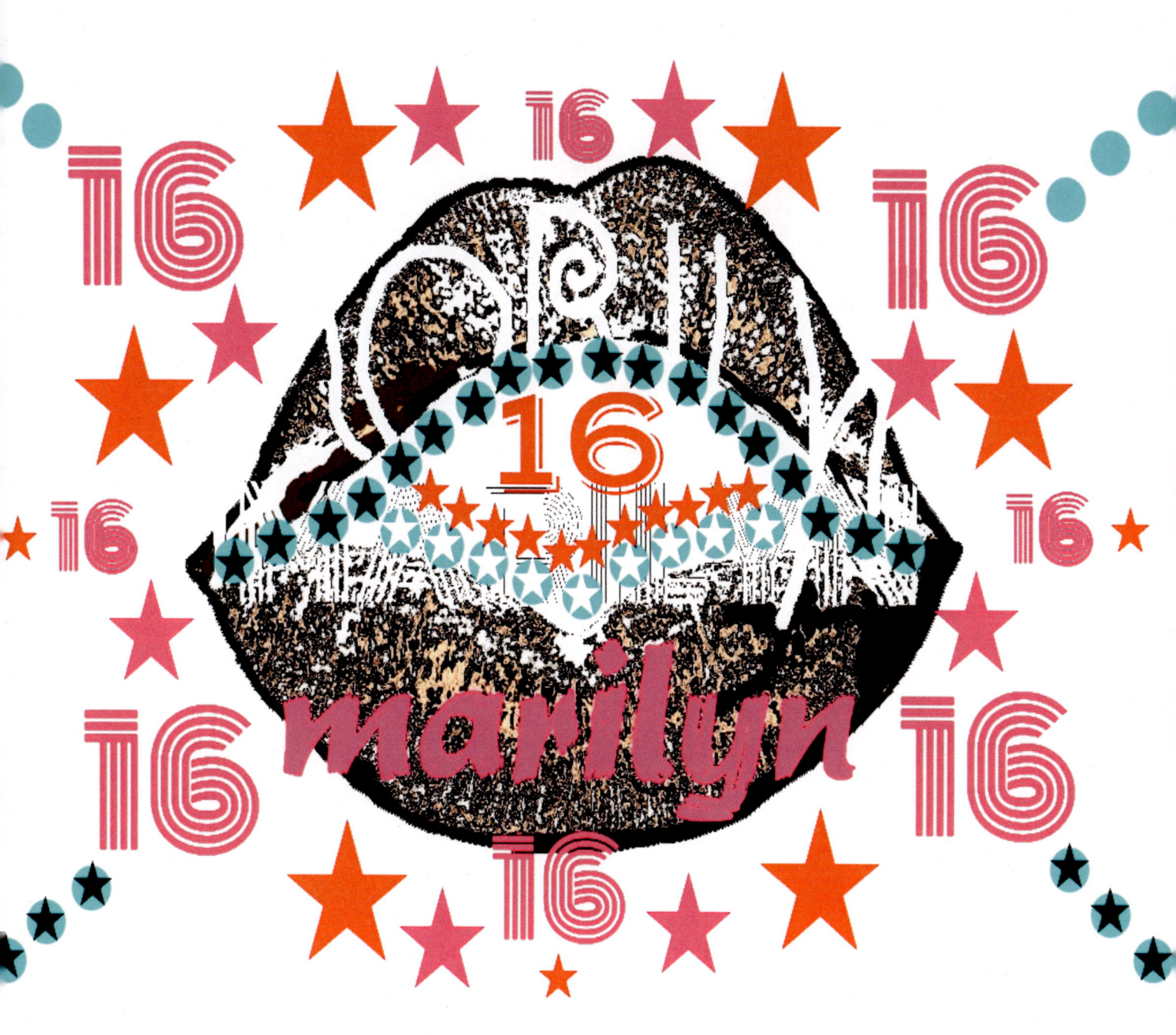

Full spiritual INTENT of our Creator's laws and judgments, inner voice strong intuition. Writers, actors and comedians. Writers, natural healers, actors, comedians. Love deeply and passionately Strong-willed good researchers very devoted, net change, good lover's true friend's strong personality, generous, value their independence sentimental, no melodrama. over-powering, philosophical, spiritual, feels a foreigner, the world of spirit. Effectively, analytical mind, penetrating beneath, concentration. Investigate, depth knowledge, wisdom. Becoming aloof, Bitterness. Impractical, Intuition. Metaphysics. Mathematic vision

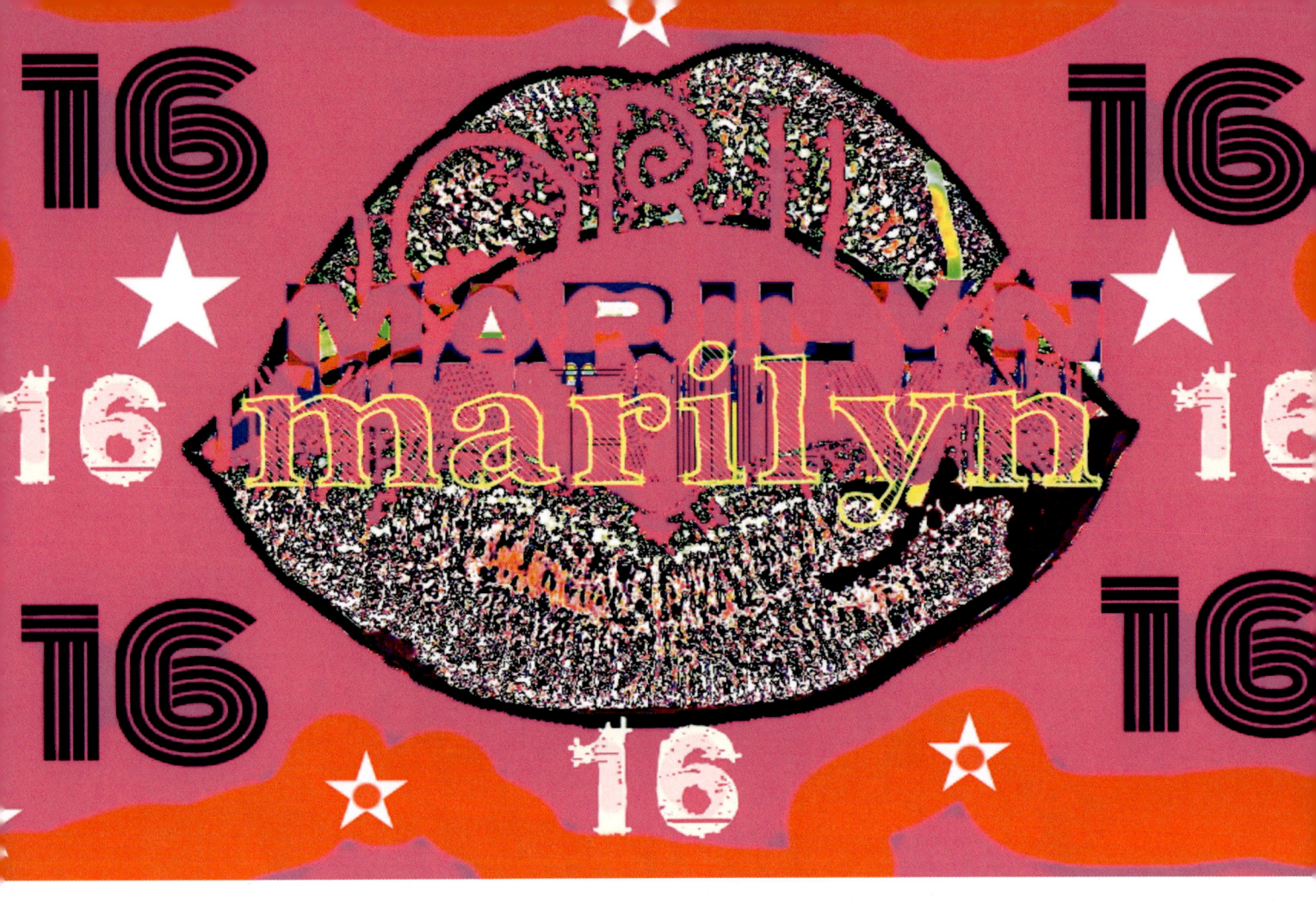

Into your story of hell and fears, I am coming with a bunch of magic keys

Taking you out of the chains of your darkness. Helping you get back to the gates of hope

Gritting my teeth while I am climbing on your heavy rocks

That had gathered on the side of your volcanic eruption

Which had closed my path into your heart, blocked the openings to your soul
Love. Let me kick the balls of your divinity.

Have me stand fully naked in front of your pet for eternity.

Put back parts of your soul into their place
Caress your naked body, since I never left you, I had never gone too far

I will sit beside you, hear your quiet breath, while you are half asleep

When your shadow becomes illuminated by the sixteen rays of light

I will gain for you a sign of a new beginning. A new beginning for me and you.

Seventeen

Jackie fans - a spell murder VER 2

Mr. President. John and I were soul mate. We knew it, as well Jacqueline was aware of it. We share the same face shape, same internal power, same mind, brain, and soul. Same targets. I never felt with any other men, the love and internal unity I felt with John, we were like twins, I felt I am melting inside of him, as if God penetrating my soul, looking at me toward his magnetic eyes. His divinity, powers, combining with mine. Any borders between us didn't last, but reality slapped on our face, each time after making a wild sex. The fact we died one after the other, shows we were a unit soul mate. I felt extremely difficult to exist without John presence. It's been for me like living with no oxygen. Why God, you don't let me live with my soul mate?

When we make love one day. John holds my face between his hands, looked deep into my eyes and said: Marilyn, you and I are two sides of the same coin, I will one day create a coin, along one side of it, I will lay your beautiful face, on the other I will put mine. Mr. president. Each time, when we had the chance to be together, we used to play like two kids inside of the garden. There were none happier people in the whole world, as me and John were, at that instant of time. Shining from glory. Cheerful, we were not afraid to be stupid, do silly things, full with laughter. We didn't want to grow up, we played like kids do. I used to make silly faces to make John laugh, I liked to jump on him, tickling him all over his body. Like children do. Then, things started to get complicated, when John got a threat on his life from the secret groups. They demand from us to break our relationship. I believe Jacqueline, was connected inside of these groups, they strain to protect her, redeem her good name and marriage. In April 27, 1961 John made his lecture about these groups. I have as well a connection inside of this society, but I was not aware of it fully, these people I am connected and meeting with, are belong to this group John was against, since, they kept it in secrets from me. I was not aware they are attempting to stimulate close to me, in order to receive info from me regard John.

I got as well a connection with France. I saved all of it as a secret from the public knowledge and eyes. At that period of time around the years 1958 - 1962, from the day I start being a Jew, I felt more tied to the theme of my Jewish soul and I was doing a kind of a research around it. This research was based on my deep beliefs about my past life, yes, I was already busier then around past lives investigation. I felt, I connect to the Mary Magdalena soul, I felt we had the same root of souls, I believe it was one more secret, which lead to a strong motivation to murder me at least, I reveal this secret to few people only, which I felt I can trust, which were close to, but they didn't take it too seriously.

Image 151 page 357. Seventeen. Model. Painter: Dr. Marilyn Monroe. Photographer: Ofer Frohlich

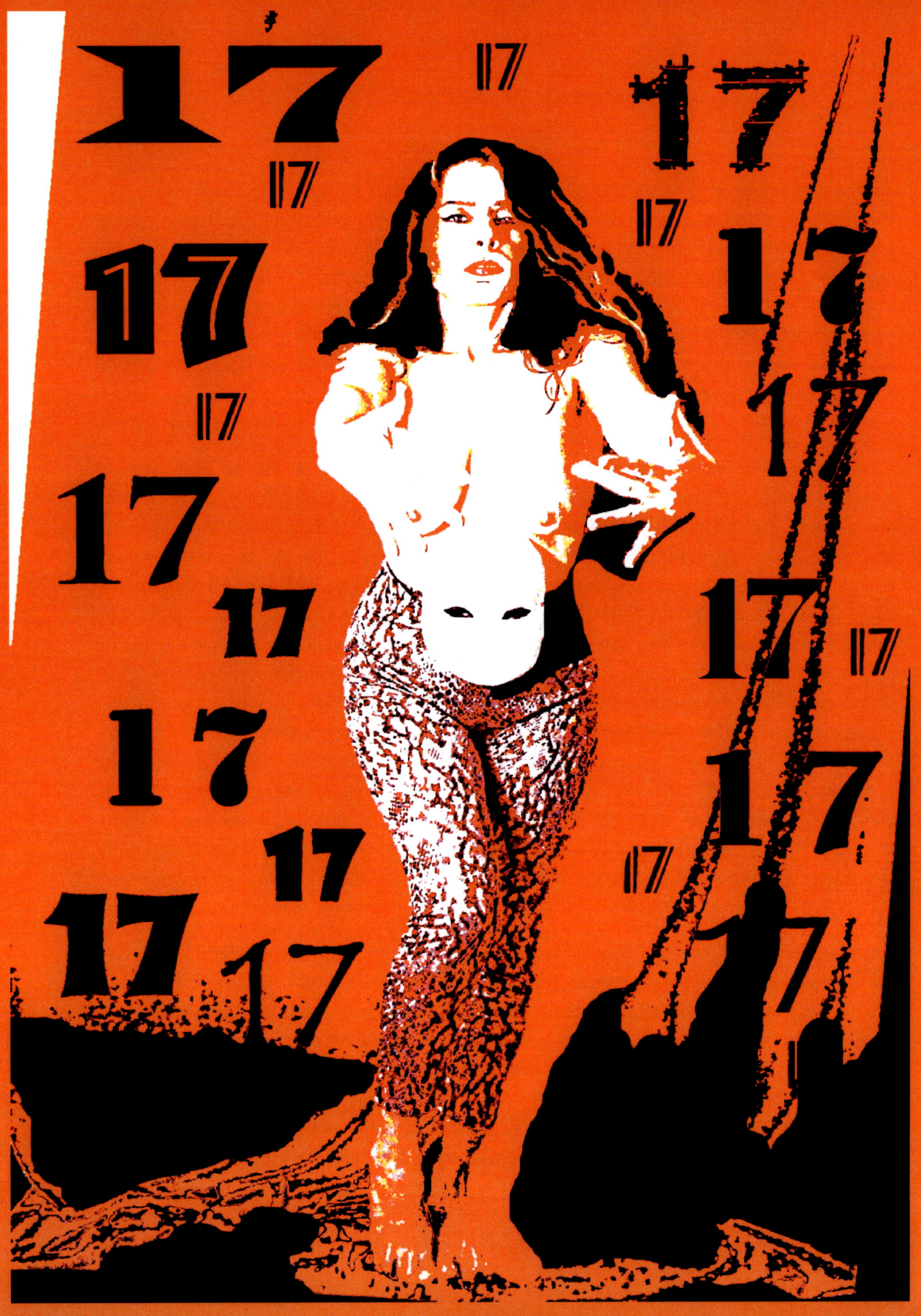
17
17
17
17
17
17
17
17
17
17
17
17
17
17
17
17
17
17
17
17
17

Obviously, in both lives, I never received the chance, to be taken extremely seriously, with my phenomenal knowledge and brain. This spot, is one of my biggest soul ache in both lives. You see, people just couldn't stand, to see me having more than what I already got. For them, my outstanding shape, was already too much to have, they could not afford, to respect my brain, it could kill them from envy and jealously. I was fully aware of it along my past life as well at the present. I attempted my best to reduce this jealousy by spreading everything I got, give it to humanity, share with them, my talents, my good will, my support, my unlimited love, but, they had abused it. I tried to lower myself as much as possible, in order to be equal to them, and have them feel natural secure side by side with me, I didn't let myself be more than the poorest human, I kept reduce myself, into the ground, just in order to fit into humanity standard around me. But It didn't help much, they had to steal and reduce anything I got, even my skin, as they did in my past by buried me. They had to kill me, in order to lower the level of jealousy they were sick with. My belief, I am part of the Mary Magdalena roots of soul, made them worry, I will become too precious for the public, "a saint". Not just a "sex symbol". They were afraid, people will want to start to obey me. I will eventually will gain, the power to rule the world. Mr. president. What could take place around the world if I was kept being alive? Can you imagine, if I was chosen to be married to the president John F. Kennedy. And bring with him, children? If I could reveal and proves the fact, I am a close source of Jesus soul and Mary Magdalena family tree. If I could find prove I am Marilyn Monroe, the living reincarnated soul of Mary Magdalena, Jesus wife. Do you understand how much powers I could gain? Do you understand why they had to murder me?

Instead, in every generation there is "a witch" who must raise on the stake. In this generation, 1962. I was chosen by these secret groups to be the witch: "To be or not to be, this is all the questions". But for me, it was: "To be Marilyn Monroe or not to be Marilyn, this was all the questions". Inside of our love affair, both me and John Kennedy, were very naïve. Apparently, Jackie, was a very strong figure, her powers were not less than John, she got groups of followers and fans, and an army of men and women. I am not sure if John was fully cognizant, but I am sure he was, more than I do. With the knowledge, how strong Jackie was, as an underground dominant queen. The army of men, which guarded her, did not see in me the right portray of the first lady, I become their personal enemy. Fans can execute a murder. In order to save their only, lovely, beautiful, dominant queen. http://en.wikipedia.org/wiki/Jacqueline_Kennedy. Me and Jackie fighting for our lives. It was a life and death battle between two lionesses. I had the need to take her place side by side to her husband. But I never dreamed to take her life for this determination. Inside of my sub conscience, she was for me, like my mother Gladys. We were two tiger's women, inside of a big cage on the top of the world, the eyes of everyone were carried toward us, like two gladiators inside of a stage. My lack of ability to fight for my life the best I could. With the same wisdom and ways Jackie managed to, was coming from the hidden information, I got inside of my brain sub conscience, which was implanted within my DNA, toward my mother's rapist. My mother will, to make an abortion, to obtain get rid of me, to kill me as a helpless fetus. Engraving "a Tattoo with a message inside of my script of life and death", which I was living upon, this hidden internal message which controlled me, was clear and cut: You do not deserve to live, Norma Jean, you should have been dead a long time ago, it is just an about a time, until someone will take care to finish what your mother, Gladys, didn't have the courage to do. This underground massage, was the reason why I could not win, in my fight with Jackie, over the kingly crown. I simply programmed to lose. My immune system didn't program to defend itself, against attacks, by the hand of another strong woman. My mother, Gladys, insane attack toward me, when I was a little kid, left my immune system full with hollows. Toward these holes, whatever other strong women, which was resemble to my mother, or reminded me of her in any path, could fetch a free entry into my life, into my soul and hurts me. The miserable outcome of it was, an undeniable attraction I felt toward their fire, the same attraction, I contracted to my mother. Like a butterfly I was flying straight toward the fire, to burned my wings. Jackie and John Kennedys as a couple, attacked me in the same manner, remind me of my mother, Gladys and my unknown father's manipulations made around my fertilization as a fetus, and a birth as an infant. Finally, I didn't measure how far Jackie will go, and John will follow her steps. Today, I am more than convinced, an extra strength behind Jackie, were used against me, in parliamentary procedure to do all kinds of spells around me, which were part of the tool to progress my death. I am not sure how much you are aware of the power of the spell methods, its ability to change the course of time and damage life. Today, I am familiar with it, since I had to learn to protect myself against it, over and over again. People are using is against me all the time. What else they can do against a very strong woman, they want to win over.

Using a spell is the easiest means, with no evidence left behind, which exit the criminal free forever. Without the power to judge him for using this method, as should. Since a spell, can wipe out not less than any other weapon you are intimate with. It can ruin anything you experienced in your life, take from you anything you had built, destroy ahead any step you will do, it can make you lose your reason, put you under a half dead, half alive existence, condemned, anything you will touch will fail. People unconscious, will feel you are contaminated with a spell, and will run away from you. It can make you take your life in your hand, it can make you be murdered by others, or simply lose the ability to life, since you will lose the will to eat, gradually you will die. Did you happen to witness this feeling on yourself? If you did, you had been contaminated with a spell, it's very similar to the Aids contamination, with one differentiate: the contamination by a spell is happening in the soul level, it caught inside anything you will touch or do, it will change your mental, emotional behavior. It doesn't contain a microbe, as the Aids does, but the ability to kill and destroy the body will be similar. With one big difference: You will not find any physical evidence, behind the murder, the cause behind death will stay hidden forever.

Image 152 page 360. Seventeen ver 2. Model. Painter: Dr. Marilyn Monroe. Photographer: Ofer Frohlich

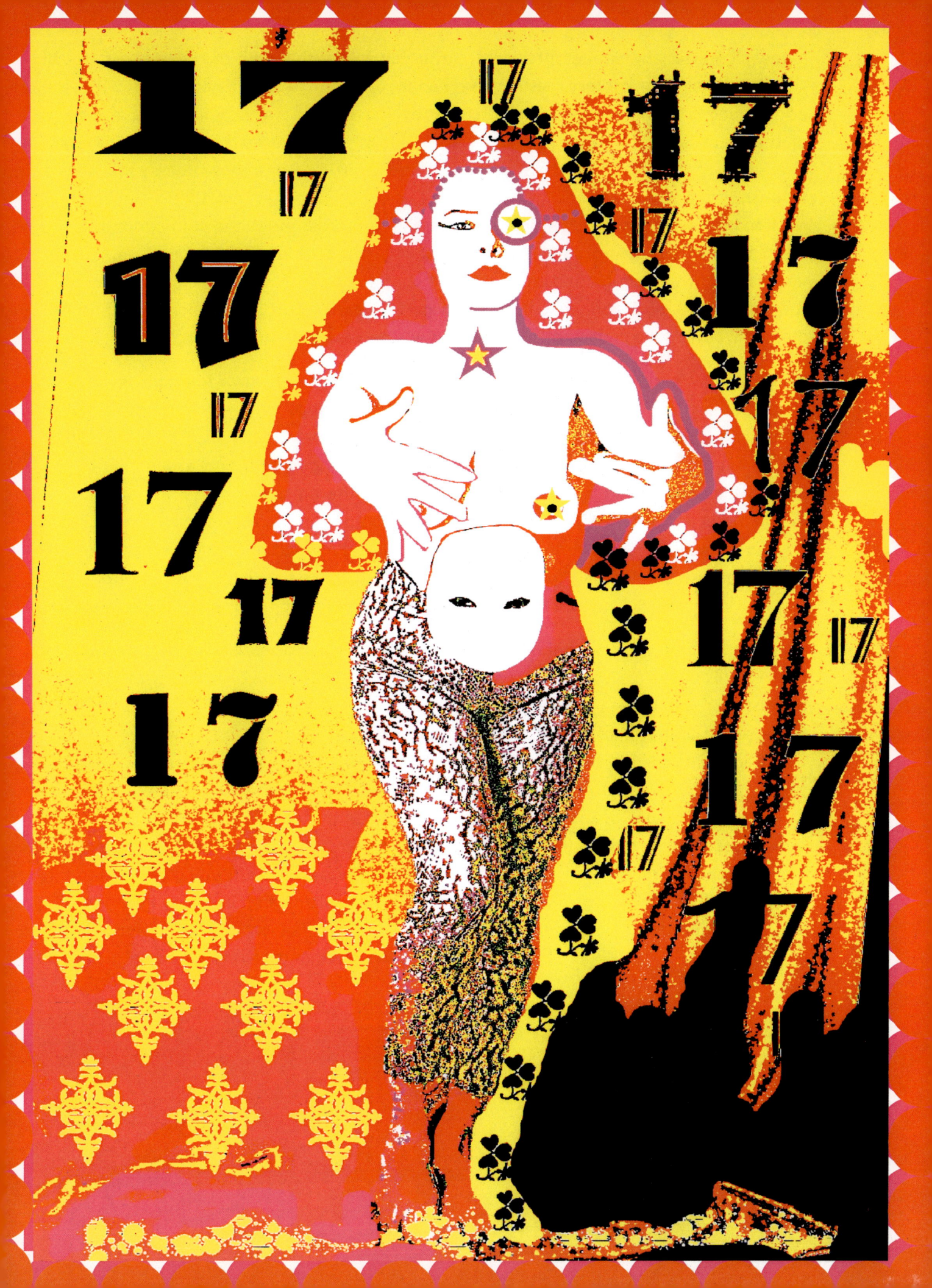

It doesn't matter how supper intelligent, clever you are, genius, with the higher IQ in the all world. If you got endless certificates hangs on your walls. If someone with the acknowledges around spells. Decided to destroy you, bury you alive, you can be at the top of the fame, and the game and you will lose it all. Plus, you will lose your life. I am guaranteeing today, and cognizant of the fact, the concluding component of my life, was as an upshot of a Jackie fans spell, whether she knew it or not. They had done a spell around my head to save her place, it's clear and cut, like the rarest, clear and cut diamond. Along the time I was meeting John, I was young, my mind didn't coop to endure or fully understand, what I am getting into. I was not open to endure the true facts, I was for John, the best sex & soul connection he could get on earth, nurtured him in any possible direction, as if I got a magical stick. https://en.wikipedia.org/wiki/Black_magic

Any men that spend time with me on earth, felt that way. I know how to match any one as a hand to a glove. John, was not failing to risk his marriage, family orientation, parents, brothers and kids or his lucrative office, for the sake of being with me. I didn't expect of him to jump on our train to heaven right away, I was going really slowly around it, nothing was an instant pudding in my life as it looks like in the outside observer, by my outside look. I did expect me and John to be eventually together, in the ascertaining kind of time. Of course I was naïve. No matter how much John loved me, felt perfectly comfortable with me, felt a truth passionately toward me. When it gets to the final cut, I was left outside his doorstep. Me, his only queen of body and soul as he named me.

My place next to him was an illusion, belong to some Fairy Stories, not to the reality world. He was fully aware of it, I was not. I always used to say: Little girls being fed with too many fairy stories which can't be performed in reality. When we, the little girls, are trying to achieve this platform of perfect love and life, as we read in the story, we failed. A big question laying behind my attitude around the Kennedys; why did I have to break my teeth, fall in love with married men, one after the other, {in both lives in a raw} which will never break the spell of the marriage for me. It doesn't refer to my IQ level which was in both cases definitely very high. Most horrifying part in this fact was the fact, these spells had continued to run around me into the present, this very same attitude continued to run after my tail. Under the same kind of fantasy. I will gain it all. When in reality I was losing it all, time after time. How many times a girl needs to fall on her butt. And doesn't comprehend, what these men are after......??????

Number Seventeen - 17 meanings

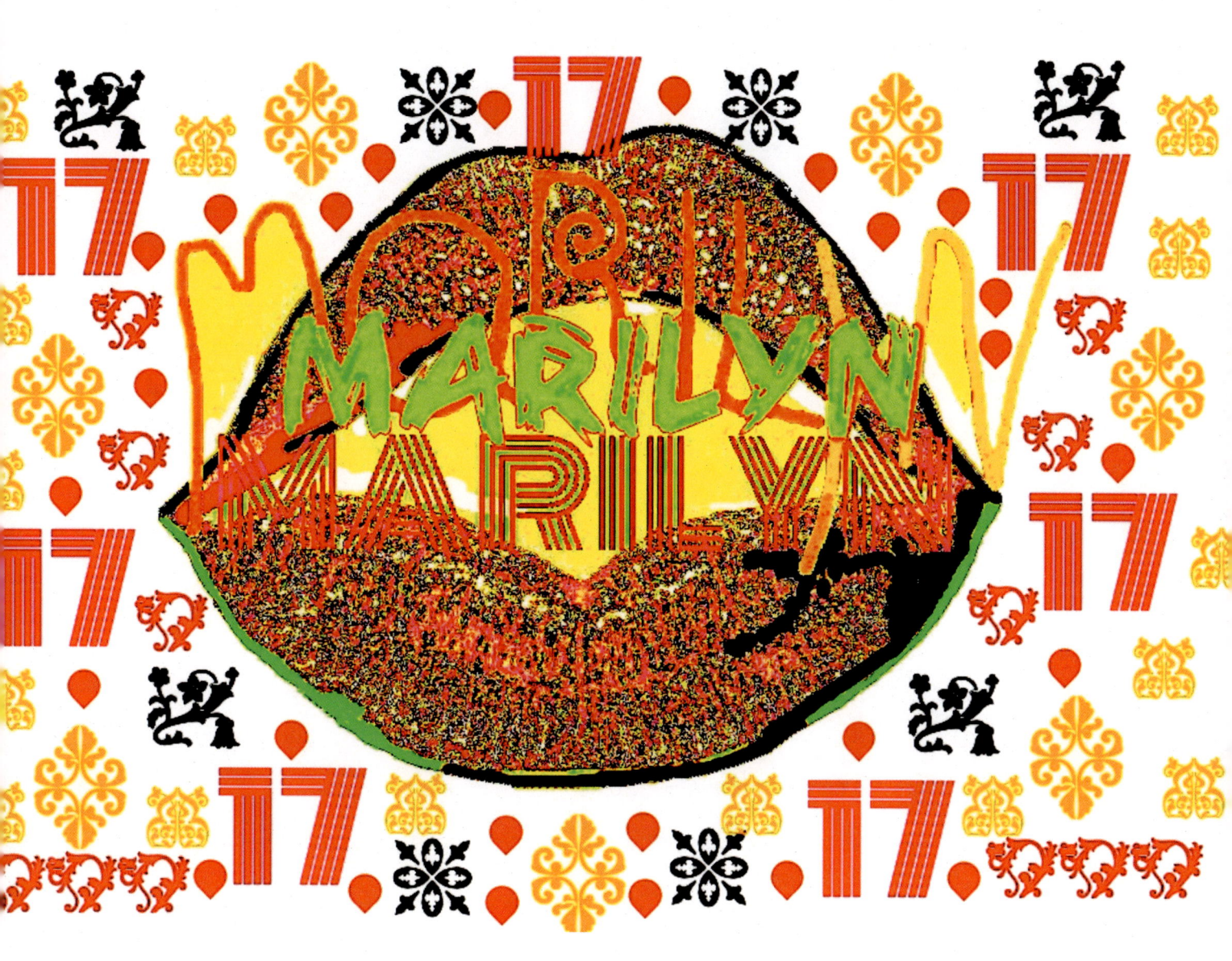

Overcoming the enemy, complete victory, Jesus Christ gained a victory over death, near sunset on Nisan 17. Greatest gift. Miraculous brought back to life. Love, Peace, promises psychic and clairvoyant, immortality. Truth and understanding hardworking Efficient. Relationships confidence a born hero a great leader takes risks, wealthy, white sheets Actors, politicians, property moguls, business. Self-determined. Self-sufficient, intuitive, spiritual and real. Entrepreneurs. The Tarot 17 card is the Stars. Wishes will come true. Chlorine atomic number. Righteousness. First gleam of dawn. Destiny. Faith with the lord within.

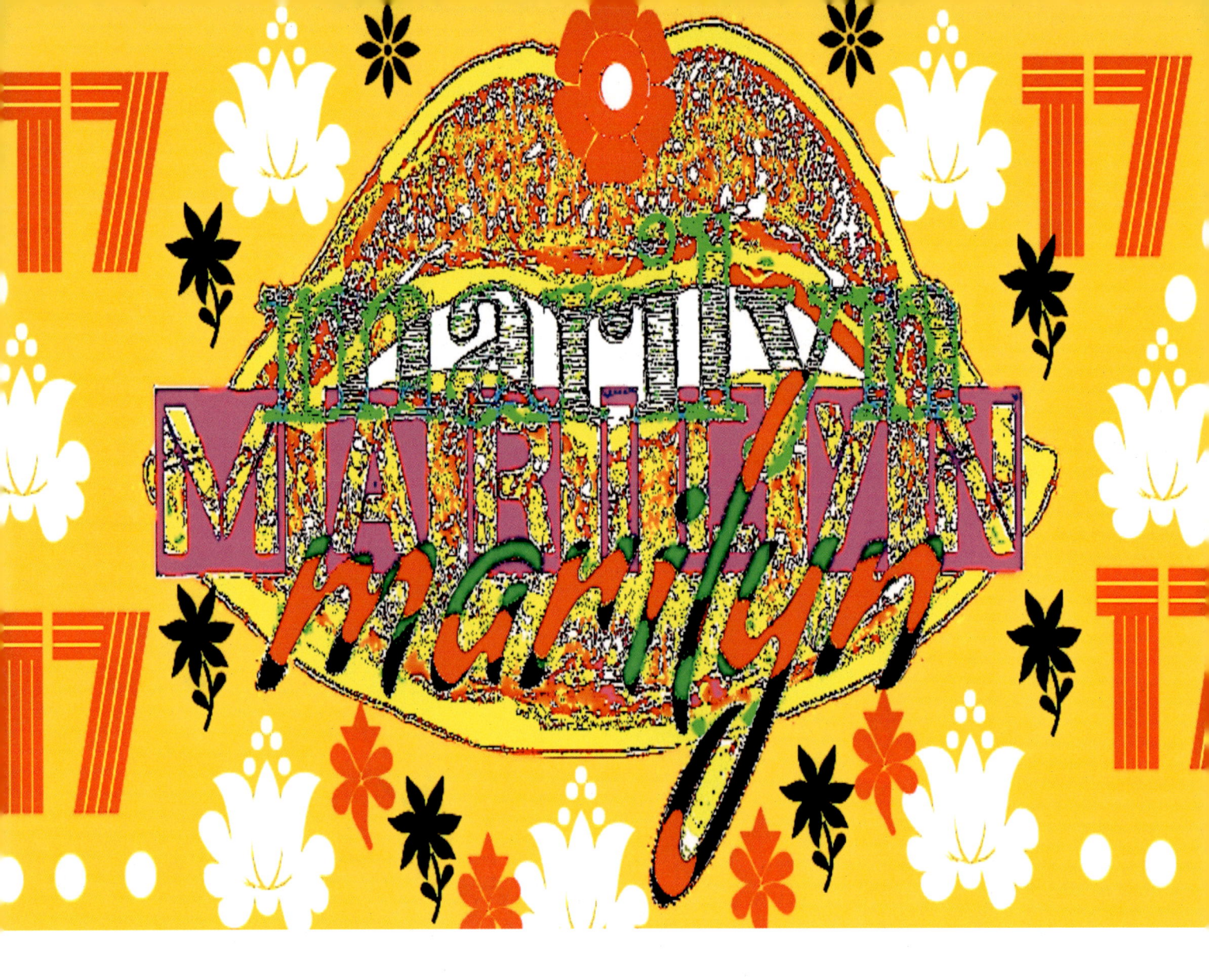

You disappeared into the infinite inner of my soul

Breaks and re-establishing old consciousness particles out of me

Destroying every part or trace, which divides my heart into seventeen parts

Destroys all the choked, and torn trace.

Source of repressed pains, resting inside of my path

Help me vomit the crush of stone out of me. Throw up barriers emotions within me

Sending me back into my virgin land of purity, my virgin plot

Cut, slits, open bursts of hope, toward my veins.

Toward the endless madness and wild torments

We had suffered from the day our soul being apart. During the big bang

THANK YOU VERY MUCH FOR READING THE THIRD SERIAL BOOK

PLEASE WRITE TO ME YOUR IMPRESSION.

AT THE THIRD AND FOURTH BOOK YOU ARE EXPOSE TO 6 MURDER SCNE

CAN YOU RECOGNIZE THE TRUE MURDER SCENE AMONG THEM?

https://www.amazon.com/author/monroemarilyn

Dr. Marilyn Monroe. Webs. Contact info:

1. Dr. Marilyn Stage 32: https://www.stage32.com/profile/120961/norma-jean-daniel

2. Dr. Marilyn Art paintings Gallery: http://drditadaniel.wix.com/normagallery

3. Dr. Marilyn cure healing web: drnorma.wix.com/cure

4. Dr. Marilyn Monroe you tube, Acting, dancing, singing, stands up

https://www.youtube.com/playlist?list=PLvtTM8NgD-yz97c0rJOIX6H3a50dsfoWv

5. Dr. Marilyn Monroe comes back LinkedIn pages: LinkedIn: http://lnkd.in/xqNJ2y

6. Dr. Marilyn Video acting photo web: http://drnorma.wix.com/dr-norma-arts

7. Dr. Marilyn Video acting web: http://drnorma.wix.com/drnorma-art

8. Linden: http://lnkd.in/bTBtceR

9. Instagram: https://www.instagram.com/dr.marilyn.monroe/

10. Dr. Marilyn Monroe email: drnormajean@gmail.com

DR MARILYN MONROE COMEBACK 2016

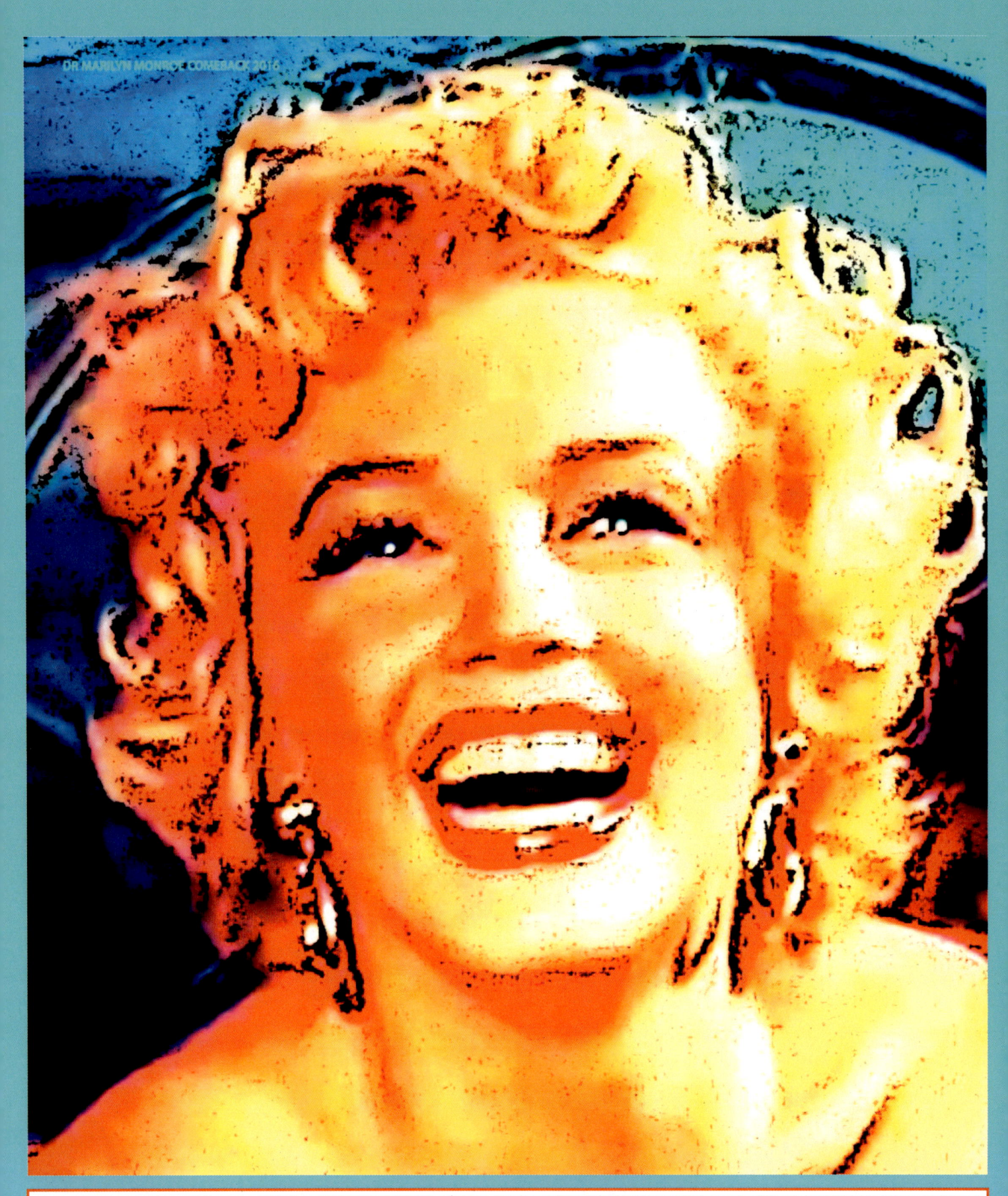

You and I together are going to bring me back to life. Against all the devilish action made by my murderers at the 5 August 1962. I truly believe we can do it. But first. You need to know better about my present life. Dr. Marilyn.

REVIEWS ON THE ANY ANGLES SERIAL BOOKS

The serial numbers of all the books were changes at the process of re-editing. Here are some reviews ahead to the changes.

The nude paintings, birthday cards book
At the paper print is volumes is seven serial book
Reviews by Mr. Grady Harp - 4 stars

This book is a delight! on first glancing at the promo material it would seem that the book's obsession with the wholly unique Hollywood icon Marilyn Monroe is a bit out of left field, but forget those safeguards to thinking scientifically and go along with the joy of the book (pictures only!) and enjoy!

The PR states, Dr. Marilyn Monroe Honorary PhD. MBMD DAM in alternative medicine, a master in arts, was found to be a Marilyn Monroe soul reborn, living in the present by the known researchers, Dr. Bruce Goldberg, conductor of the clinic in California and an internationally renowned expert in hypnosis and the study of past lives through hypnosis. In this series of books in the name "Any angel has the right to live twice" Dr. Marilyn that was reborn 3 years after her death that took place on August 5, 1962.'

Or to quote from Marilyn herself, 'In this book I will reveal to you a little more sign of the fact I am Marilyn Monroe. My artistic creation describes from the first day I start to draw as a child at this present lifetime my former life unsolved issue, just about my mysterious death and life. This is an artistic creation. For me the meaning of art is the action of pouring your soul into some piece of material. Letting this material have inside of it your stamp. I think that if you will but let yourself co it. You will find out of all world hiding there inside and inside of your soul'. [sic]

It is unclear in what language this book originated but an editor would be very helpful in making it more readable. The art is photographic and painted and multimedia in nature – all in hot wild colors. For those who love pop art this is a bonus. And the book is definitely one to be taken as it is offered – an homage to a great entertainment figure of our history. Grady Harp, July 16

The cure book

Mr. Grady Harp - 5 stars

This book at the paper print is volumes fifth and six serial books.

For those unfamiliar with this series of books, this set of four volumes deals with the return to life of Marilyn Monroe. While some of the later volumes deal with issues this book is far more accessible in that it is truly the flavor of the Hollywood Icon, still among us!

This volume 2 of the four series differs from the other art focused books in that Dr Monroe includes Principles for the Protection of Health (Kidney protection, medicine/poison/drugs/alcohol, Nutrition and Cleansing, the dangers of salt, the importance of Sleep, protecting the immune system, knowing your sexuality life energy core), her resume, poems, songs, package card games, paintings to remove form the book and hang on the wall, and a Petition for the opening of the investigation of the Marilyn Monroe Murder Case.
There are still many images of the star – manipulated photographs which are based on images by the photographers made dramatically colorful by Dr Monroe.
The series is fascinating and worth viewing and we can only hope that the rebirth of Marilyn Monroe is a possibility! Grady Harp, July 16

The self- portrait book

Mr. Grady Harp - 5 stars

This book at the paper print is volume no eight.

This fourth book in a series is an absolute delight! On first glancing at the promo material it would seem that this book's obsession with the wholly unique Hollywood icon Marilyn Monroe is a bit out of left field, but forget those safeguards to thinking scientifically and go along with the joy of the book (pictures only!) and enjoy!

There are four volumes in this set, each written by Dr. Marilyn Monroe – this book is Volume 4 and is completely composed of art – various thoughts and views of beloved images of Marilyn Monroe. To help the reader understand the project, the PR states, 'Dr. Marilyn Monroe Honorary PhD. MBMD DAM in alternative medicine, a master in arts, was found to be a Marilyn Monroe soul reborn, living in the present by the known researchers, Dr. Bruce Goldberg, conductor of the clinic in California and an internationally renowned expert in hypnosis and the study of past lives through hypnosis. In this series of books in the name "Any angel has the right to live twice" Dr. Marilyn that was reborn 3 years after her death that took place on August 5, 1962.'

Or to quote from Marilyn herself, 'In this book I will reveal to you a little more sign of the fact I am Marilyn Monroe. My artistic creation describes from the first day I start to draw as a child at this present lifetime my former life unsolved issue, just about my mysterious death and life. This is an artistic creation. For me the meaning of art is the action of pouring your soul into some piece of material. Letting this material have inside of it your stamp. I think that if you will but let yourself co it. You will find out of all world hiding there inside and inside of your soul'. [sic]

I will be happy to see your

High ranking, positive reviews of my books. Please send your review after publish it to drnormajean@gmail.com to get one more book at the serial in kindle for free. And a thank you letter sign by me. Add your review just below each book

https://amzn.com/B01HFQCVIK

https://amzn.com/B01H4AEFAE

More About the Author

› Visit Amazon's Dr. Marilyn Monroe Page

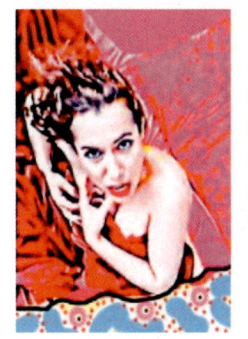

Biography

Dr. Marilyn Monroe. an Honorary. PhD. MBMD. DAM in alternative medicine. A master in arts, was found by the internationally renowned expert in hypnosis and the study of past lives through hypnosis. To be a Marilyn Monroe Indications, in an infinite act of previous life continuity of Marilyn Monroe and similarities in all scopes of life with Marilyn Monroe. In this series of books in the name "Any angel has the right to live twice" Dr. Marilyn that was re testimony around her past life and death. You will fall out of your hair while reading this book. This extreme new case. Ahead in this series of book, Dr. Marilyn published the first volume "white secrets". That had won the sup years ago in 2002. In this book. Norma broke the silence borders on topics that used to downplay the speech in

Show More

✓ Following

Customer Reviews

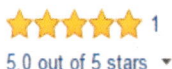

★★★★★ 1
5.0 out of 5 stars ▼

5 star	████████	100%
4 star		0%
3 star		0%
2 star		0%
1 star		0%

Share your thoughts with other customers

[Write a customer review]

See the customer review ›

Top Customer Reviews

★★★★★ **Marilyn Monroe Reborn in art**

By Grady Harp HALL OF FAME TOP 100 REVIEWER VINE VOICE on July 2, 2016

Format: Kindle Edition | Verified Purchase

This fourth book in a series is an absolute delight! On first glancing at the promo material it would seem that this book's obsession with the wholly unique Hollywood icon Marilyn Monroe is a bit out of left field, but forget those safeguards to thinking scientifically and go along with the joy of the book (pictures only!) and enjoy!

There are four volumes in this set, each written by Dr Marilyn Monroe – this book is Volume 4 and is completely composed of art – various thoughts and views of beloved images of Marilyn Monroe. To help the reader understand the project, the PR states, 'Dr. Marilyn Monroe Honorary PhD. MBMD DAM in alternative medicine, a master in arts, was found to be a Marilyn Monroe soul reborn, living in the present by the known researchers. Dr. Bruce Goldberg, conductor of the clinic in California and an internationally renowned expert in hypnosis and the study of

A petition for the benefit of the opening of

The investigation murder case of Marilyn Monroe

This investigation is about the human right of Marilyn Monroe soul, whatever you believe or not yet have the facts that will be your key and took to understand, I am Marilyn at my present. Without your help this Pandora box around my past murder is going to stay buried underground You can help by a few simple actions to change it, and take the power back from my murdered

1. Send a letter, to the president of the USA. why it's important, to investigate this case

2. if you send me a copy of your letter, I will exhibit it together with other letters at the voice of Marilyn fans future book. your letter should carry your full truth name. The city and country you are living in. Please send your letter drnormajean@gmail.com.

3. subscribe on the petition below. I had never published it; you may be the first to sign.

4. If you want to manage one of my Facebook groups. Let me know at the same email.

http://www.ipetitions.com/petition/marilyn-monroe-open-a-police-investigation

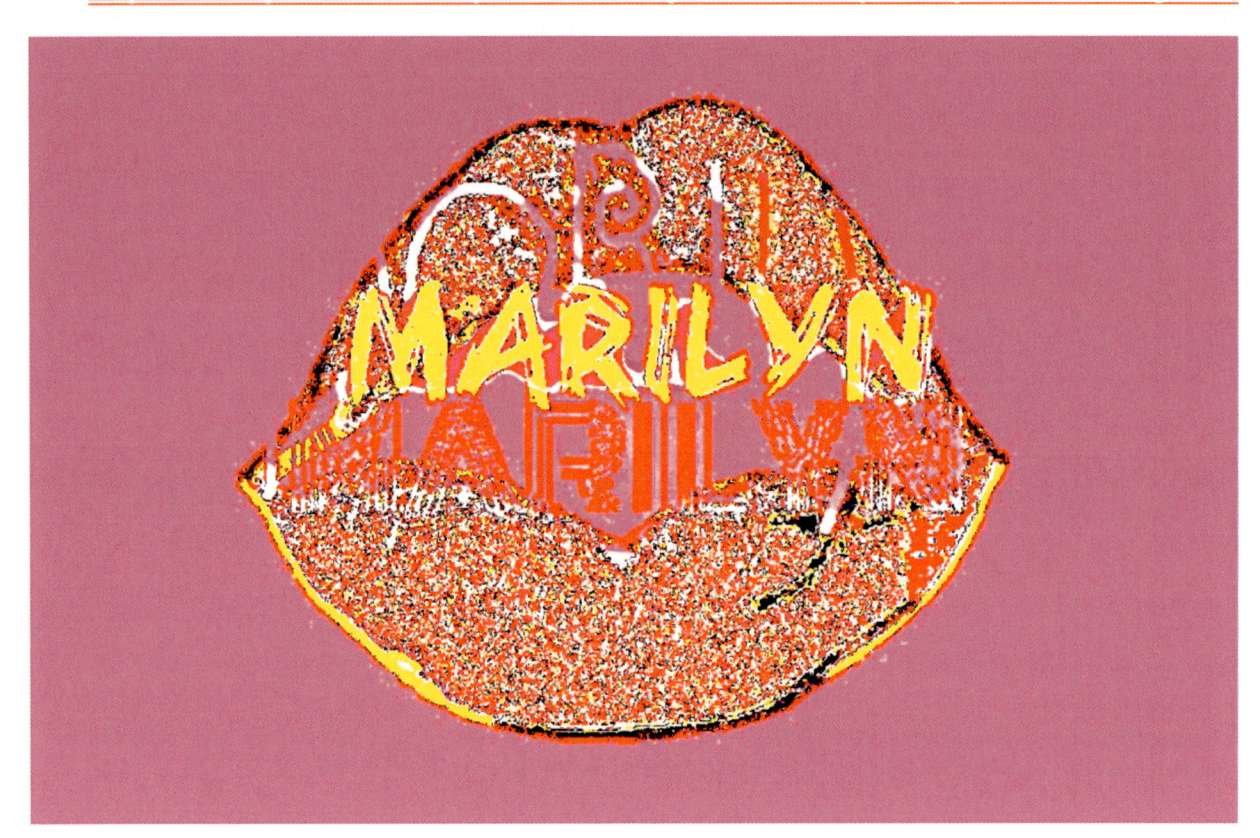

Thank you God bless

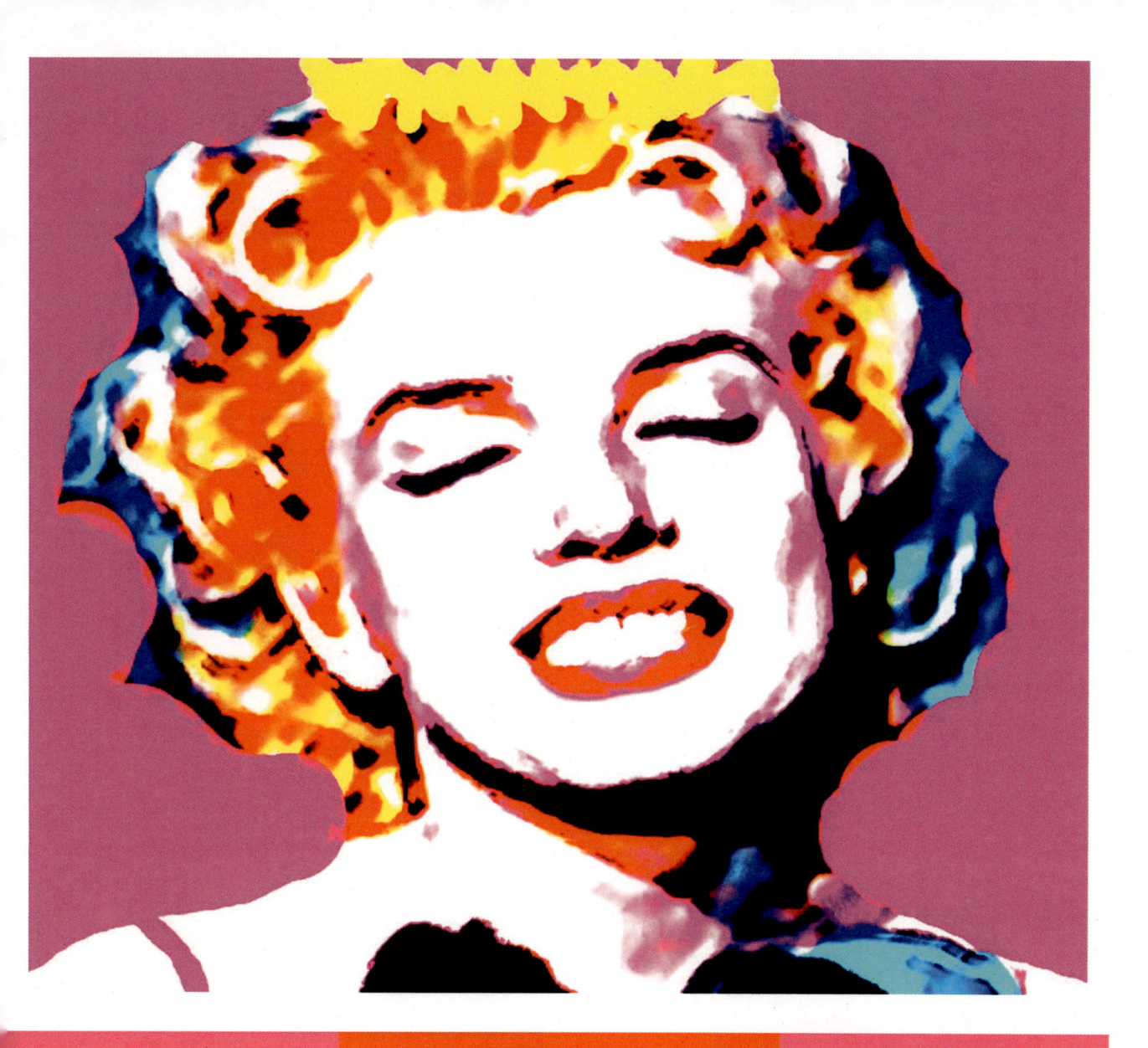

Thank you

From the

Bottom of my heart

Dr. Marilyn Monroe

Made in the USA
Monee, IL
06 March 2022